HIV, Health, and Your Community

A Guide for Action

This book is dedicated to the many people throughout the world who face the challenge of working and living with HIV every day.

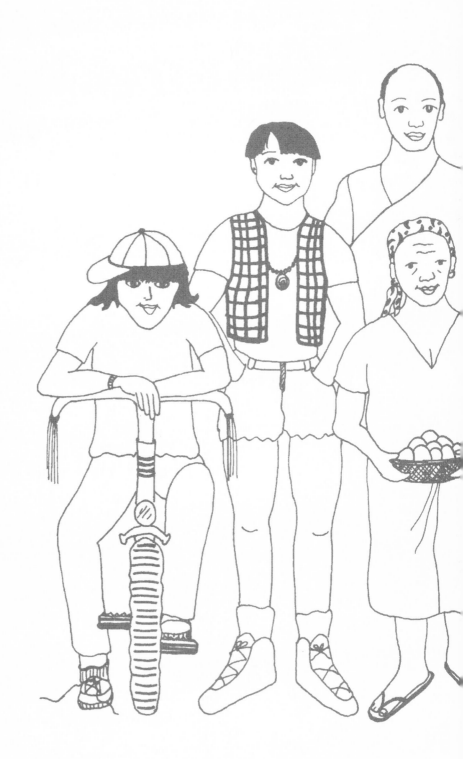

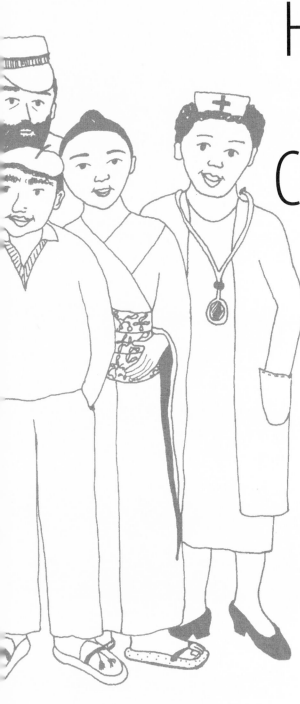

HIV, Health, and Your Community

A Guide for Action

Reuben Granich, M.D., M.P.H.
Jonathan Mermin, M.D., M.P.H.

Illustrations by
Mona Sfeir

With contributions by
Suzan Goodman, M.D.

THE HESPERIAN FOUNDATION
Berkeley, California, USA

Library of Congress Cataloging-in-Publication Data

Granich, Reuben, 1963–
    HIV, health, and your community : a guide for action /
Reuben Granich, Jonathan Mermin ; with contributions
by Suzan Goodman ; illustrations by Mona Sfeir.
        p.   cm.
    ISBN 0-942364-40-6
(paper)
        1. AIDS (Disease)   2. Community health aides.
I. Mermin, Jonathan, 1965– .   II. Title.
RC607.A26G626   1999
362.1'969792—DC21   99-12967

Original printing 1999
Fourth printing 2006

Book design by Mark Ong

With your help, this book can be updated and improved.
Please send any comments, criticisms or suggestions to:

The Hesperian Foundation
1919 Addison Street, #304
Berkeley, California 94704 USA
e-mail: hesperian@hesperian.org
website: www.hesperian.org

Printed in the United States of America

Contents

Acknowledgments

Many people gave their time, energy, and a small part of their souls to this book. Mona Sfeir patiently provided advice and encouragement as well as creative illustrations. Rebecca Bunnell reminded us of our labor's purpose and gave invaluable comments based on years of experience in the field. As clinician, teacher, and community activist, S. Ira Greene, our mentor in medical school, exemplified qualities we wished to see more of in ourselves. Throughout the years he provided unflagging encouragement and advice, and he is dearly missed. Larry Peiperl graciously and insightfully reviewed clinical aspects of the text. Robert Siegel was kind enough to edit many parts of the text, and he showed us how enthusiasm mixed with intelligence can overcome many obstacles. Susan Allen provided us with a model of what a compassionate AIDS project for women could accomplish in a turbulent environment. Pauline Keough inspired us with her work with Rwandan women, giving us insight into their everyday courage and struggle to survive. Nadia Wetzler provided critical support, and her review during a lull in our work helped us finish the manuscript. Suzan Goodman contributed to early drafts of several chapters. Alan Pont served as mentor and writing coach. Nell Mermin and Alexandra Saler steadfastly edited early drafts. Karie Youngdahl, in her charming and matter-of-fact way, edited and propelled us along. Omer Pasi shared his considerable understanding of the HIV epidemic in Zaire. Barry Schoub gave us helpful comments on an early draft of the manuscript. The administration of the Stanford Medical School, especially Patricia Cross and John Steward, gave us the time and support needed to begin the project. The Morrison Institute provided funding to assist us with the early stages of the book, and Terry Karl of the Center for Latin American Studies supported our field research. Muriel Bell at Stanford University Press was invaluable in accepting the challenge of publishing this book. No acknowledgment would be complete without recognition of Jan Spauschus Johnson and Lynn Stewart, whose thoughtful and caring editing made this book a reality. For this update by Hesperian in 2005, Fiona Thomson provided coordination, research and writing; Susan McCallister edited the revisions; Leana Rosetti, Sarah Wallis, and Iñaki Fernández de Retana did production work to fit the new material into our format; Todd Jailer proofread; and Ty Koontz updated the index.

We thank our families, friends, and coworkers for for their understanding and support.

R.G.   ·   J.M.

Introduction

The idea for this book grew out of our experiences working to help growing numbers of people with HIV (human immunodeficiency virus). In Rwanda, one of us met a doctor who struggled to care for a hospital ward overflowing with women with HIV and tuberculosis. Families were camped outside, cooking and caring for their sick relatives; patients without families suffered because food and other supplies were scarce, but often other people shared what they had. Working long days under tough conditions, the members of the health care team had to make difficult decisions about treatment. They watched as a few patients died each day despite their best efforts.

Health workers, social workers, and educators joined together to lessen the suffering caused by HIV. When asked where they had learned to do their jobs, they shrugged their shoulders and pointed to each other. They had learned from experience and word of mouth. Why was there no guide that addressed some of the basic issues regarding HIV disease in areas where most of the people with HIV live? There were thousands of scientific articles about HIV, but the language in them was often obscure and the topics not relevant. In addition, these articles were often unavailable to health care workers in the less industrialized world. What was missing was a comprehensive reference book covering basic topics related to the HIV epidemic.

We have tried to write a book that is both readable and practical. We describe some of the experiences of people we have known, many of whom have died from HIV or in the civil disturbances that frequently accompany the epidemic. Bearing in mind our readers—local health and community workers who have a desire to learn more about HIV—we have tried to keep the language and format simple.

The book is meant for people who are searching for answers to questions about HIV prevention, epidemiology, diagnosis, and treatment. Each chapter begins with a fictional story; where useful, boxes with text or illustrations have been added to highlight key points. At the end of each chapter we answer questions raised by the story, hoping at the same time to answer some of the reader's questions. The appendix discusses common diseases suffered by people with HIV and treatments for them. It is intended for the doctor or nurse who is involved in caring for people with HIV disease, and unlike the other chapters requires some basic medical knowledge. HIV health care is always changing, and some of the recommendations in the chapter may be outdated. Adaptations to individual situations are encouraged. Finally, we have included a glossary of words often used in discussions about HIV.

In Chapter 1 we meet Shoba, a student from Pakistan. We learn about the basics of HIV biology and how HIV affects a person's immune system, the nature of a virus, why viruses are difficult to treat, and the difference between HIV-1 and HIV-2. We explain the basic elements of the immune system, focusing on the cells most affected by HIV. We end the chapter with a short discussion of medicines against HIV.

In Chapter 2 we meet Saleema from Morocco. Saleema has a brother she thinks has signs of HIV infection. We explain some of the symptoms that someone with HIV may experience.

In Chapters 3 and 4 we meet Min-Soo from South Korea and Lon Chin from China. Min-Soo asks questions about where AIDS (acquired immune deficiency syndrome) was first found, how we know HIV is not spread by mosquitoes, and how to figure out how many people have HIV. We present a short history of the HIV epidemic and discuss how HIV has spread worldwide and how it interacts with other diseases. Lon Chin's parents are afraid to let her move to the United States because they think she will get AIDS. Lon Chin wants to know about how much HIV and AIDS there is in the world so that she can help her parents understand why she will not get HIV by studying in the United States. We discuss HIV and present the latest information on the number of people with HIV and AIDS.

In Chapters 5 and 6 we meet Olga from Uzbekistan and Clarence from Ghana, who are concerned about how HIV is spread from one person to another. They want to know what kinds of sex put them at risk and what other ways there are of getting HIV. We explain how HIV is spread and how it is not spread. We talk about the role of other sexually transmitted diseases in the spread of HIV and about how drugs and alcohol can increase a person's chance of getting HIV.

In Chapters 7 and 8 we meet Jean-Patrice from French Guiana and José from Mexico. Jean-Patrice wants to know how well the HIV test works. We discuss the test, the difference between confidential and anonymous testing, and the accuracy of test results. We also discuss mandatory testing, how testing relates to family planning, and how it may encourage or discourage behavior change. José is worried about how much blood is needed for the test and what he should do after he gets the results. We explain common testing procedures and pre- and post-test counseling.

In Chapter 9 we meet Odette from Gabon. Her situation is complicated. Her social standing in the community and in her family influence her chances of getting HIV. We discuss how economics, ethnicity, health care beliefs, education, drug and alcohol use, prejudice, and age can all affect a person's risk of getting HIV.

In Chapter 10 we meet Angela from Brazil. Angela is pregnant and finds out she has HIV. She is worried about telling her boyfriend and says she is thinking about killing herself. We discuss how health care workers, family members, and friends can support people who have HIV. We describe some of the challenges of coping with HIV, some basic interventions that can help people with HIV stay healthy, and the benefits of support groups, community support, and home care. We give some tips on how to avoid burning out as a caregiver.

In Chapters 11, 12, and 13 we meet Phan from Vietnam, Carlos from the United States, and María from Peru. Carlos needs help teaching others to avoid the virus. He wants to know how to approach high school students and teenagers who do not go to school. We describe places for HIV outreach and give him the tools to either start his own prevention project or help an existing project in his community. Phan needs hels and how to encourage everyone to participate. We also provide a sample lesson plan for a day-long training session. María needs help finding more funding for the project she runs for women with HIV and AIDS. We discuss ways to look for funding both in her community and outside it.

We would like to add a word of caution. HIV, AIDS, and sex are sensitive topics. Parts of our book may be offensive to you. We do not intend to shock readers, but we use explicit language throughout the book in order to bring you the most accurate information possible. You may have to change some of this language to work with your community.

We hope you find this book useful. We know it can be improved with your suggestions. We are always interested in hearing about HIV projects and people's personal experiences working in the field, and we welcome thoughts from people with HIV, their families, and caregivers. Please send your comments to us in care of the Hesperian Foundation, 1919 Addison Street # 304, Berkeley, California 94704, USA, or visit the Hesperian website at *www.hesperian.org*.

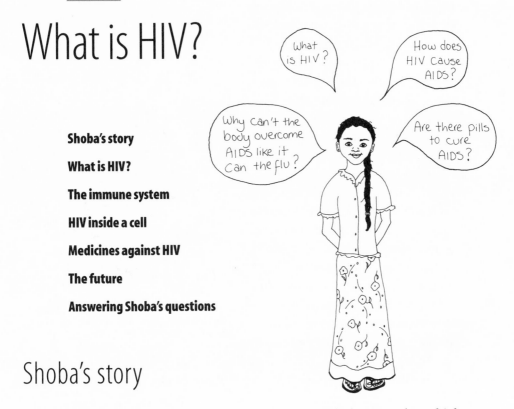

1

What is HIV?

Shoba's story

Shoba is a fifteen-year-old student in Pakistan. She has just taken a biology class. She already knew that she could prevent illness by washing her hands after going to the bathroom and before she cooks or eats. But in class, she learned about how the body defends itself against sickness. She read about AIDS and the immune system, and she is interested in learning more about HIV and its effect on the body. Someday she wants to be a health worker. Shoba comes to you and asks, "What is HIV? How does HIV cause AIDS? Why can't the body overcome AIDS like it can the flu? Are there pills to cure AIDS?"

What is HIV?

HIV stands for "human immunodeficiency virus": "human" because the virus causes disease only in people; "immunodeficiency" because the immune system, which normally protects a person from disease, becomes weak; "virus" because like all viruses, HIV is a small organism that infects living things and uses them to make copies of itself. HIV causes AIDS (acquired immune deficiency syndrome). AIDS is a group of diseases that occur when a person's immune system is damaged by HIV. Most people with HIV feel healthy for the first few years after getting the virus, but later they become sick with AIDS (see Chapter 2).

Viruses are tiny organisms, even smaller than the bacteria that cause tuberculosis or cholera. They are common—so common that we all become infected with them many times throughout our lives. Viruses cause the common cold, as well as polio, measles, mumps, and the flu. These viruses can be spread by coughing, sneezing, or touching. HIV is different. Even though it also is a virus, it cannot be spread in any of these ways. HIV can be spread only by

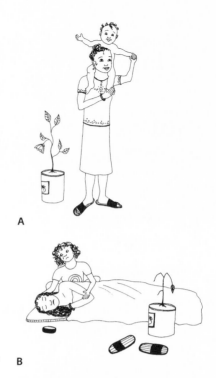

A

B

(A) Most people feel healthy for the first few years after getting HIV. (B) Later they become sick with AIDS.

certain sex acts, blood, dirty needles and other instruments, and from a mother to her unborn baby or a baby she is breastfeeding (see Chapters 5 and 6).

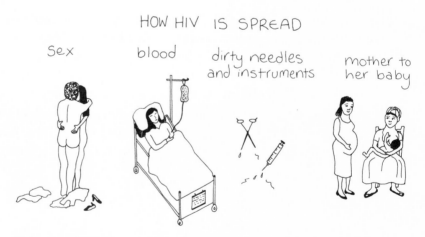

HOW HIV IS SPREAD

Sex   blood   dirty needles and instruments   mother to her baby

Viruses are difficult to treat with medicines. They are not affected by the medicines that work against bacteria; even powerful antibiotics like penicillin or tetracycline do not work against them. HIV is a special kind of virus called a retrovirus. It makes copies of itself in a different way than many other viruses; because of this, it is more difficult to treat. The best way to stop the spread of viruses and the diseases they cause is to prevent people from getting infected in the first place. You can stop the spread of viruses like measles by using a vaccine.

HIV is different because there is no vaccine for it. But changing behavior can also stop the spread of disease. For example, washing your hands after going to the bathroom will lower your chance of spreading diarrhea to other people. Changing behavior can also stop the spread of HIV.

There are two types of human immunodeficiency virus: HIV-1 and HIV-2. Like sister and brother, they have similarities and differences. HIV-1 is found in all parts of the world. HIV-2 is found mostly in West Africa. Since the spread of both viruses can be prevented in the same ways, we will discuss HIV-1 and HIV-2 together as "HIV."

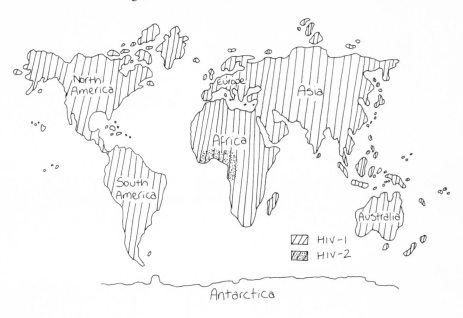

The immune system

"Immune" means safe and protected. The body's immune system works to keep out invaders such as viruses (like the one that causes polio), bacteria (like the one that causes tuberculosis), parasites (like the one that causes malaria),

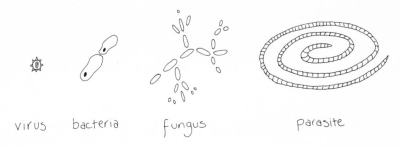

virus   bacteria   fungus   parasite

and fungi (like the one that causes yeast infections). These organisms can infect people and cause disease and death.

The immune system is made of different types of cells. Cells are tiny parts of a person's body that are too small to see without a microscope. The body is made up of billions of cells. Each type of cell plays a different role; some cells make up bone, others muscle, others the immune system.

Cells of the immune system, like most other cells in the body, have a center called a nucleus. The nucleus, or "headquarters" of the cell, contains DNA (deoxyribonucleic acid), or genes. The nucleus acts as chief of the cell and controls its activities. It tells the cell when to make a new sub-stance needed by the body or when to make another cell. For each person, the DNA in all cells is the same. Each cell uses different parts of the same DNA to lead its activities.

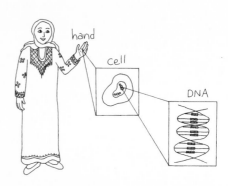

People are made up of billions of cells. Every cell contains DNA.

If the immune system meets something from outside the body, it makes small (microscopic) particles made of protein called antibodies. These stick to invaders and help the rest of the immune system find and destroy them. This allows a person to avoid illness, or to become well if already ill.

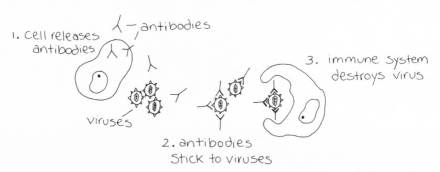

1. Cell releases antibodies — antibodies

viruses

2. antibodies stick to viruses

3. immune system destroys virus

A special protein called CD4 marks the outsides of some immune system cells, making them different from other immune cells. The CD4 marking is like the stripes that make a zebra different from a horse. CD4 cells are also called helper T cells, because the body sends them to identify and defend against invaders like viruses and bacteria. However, HIV enters cells that have CD4 on their surface. In other words, the CD4 cells are attacked by the same virus, HIV, that they are trying to defend against.

This is a serious problem, because the body needs CD4 cells to defend itself against diseases. This is why people with HIV often become sick from organisms that people without HIV can usually fight off. Bacteria, fungi, other viruses, and parasites take the "opportunity" to infect a person with a weak immune system. The illnesses they cause are called "opportunistic infections," and they can kill someone with HIV.

HIV inside a cell

When HIV gets inside the body, it looks for CD4 cells. When it finds a CD4 cell, it attaches itself to the cell and enters it. Once inside, HIV finds the DNA in the cell nucleus. HIV makes a copy of itself from DNA building materials in the cell. This copy then hides itself in the CD4 cell's DNA. Under a microscope, the cell's DNA appears normal, even though it is now mixed with HIV DNA. Once safely hidden in the cell's DNA, HIV can do one of two things. It can stay quietly in the cell, or it can turn on the cell's DNA and use the cell's machinery to make copies of itself. To make copies it uses a protein called reverse transcriptase. If it begins reproducing, it can make thousands of new HIV. These new viruses leave the cell and enter other CD4 cells and the same thing happens again. Some people think the virus makes a billion copies of itself every day.

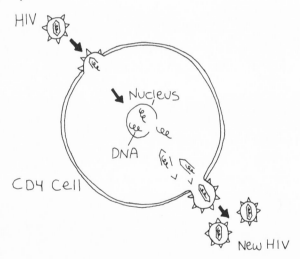

HIV enters CD4 cells and makes copies of itself.

When the HIV DNA lies inside of the cell's DNA, there is no way for the body to get rid of it. HIV hides so well that the body does not even know it is there. This ability to hide lets HIV spread within the body. In addition to making copies of itself within affected cells, HIV has another way of reproducing. When the cell decides it is time to make another cell, it reproduces HIV DNA as well as its own. Each time that a new cell is made, HIV is also made. Because there is no easy way to tell the difference between DNA from HIV and DNA from the body's cells, there are no medicines that can completely remove the virus from the body.

Medicines against HIV

People are making medicines that work against the illnesses that people get after HIV weakens their immune system. They are also looking for ways to stop HIV from reproducing, and they are trying to make vaccines that would prevent a person from getting HIV. In the Appendix we describe medicines used to treat HIV-related opportunistic infections. In this section we will discuss some medicines that work directly against HIV.

There are several types of drugs that work to stop HIV. To be effective, several drugs must be used together. These drugs given together are called antiretroviral therapy (ART). One type of drug that fights HIV is the reverse transcriptase inhibitor. Examples of this type of medicine are zidovudine (AZT), stavudine (d4T), lamivudine (3TC), nevirapine, efavirenz, and emtricitabine. Reverse transcriptase inhibitors work by stopping HIV from becoming part of the cell's DNA. Another type of drug is a protease inhibitor, such as lopinovir/ritonavir and nelfinavir. Protease inhibitors stop HIV from putting itself together and reproducing. The last type of drug for ART is called a fusion inhibitor, such as enfurvirtide, which prevents HIV from entering cells.

By slowing the ability of the virus to make copies of itself, ART is often able to keep people alive for many years. However, it cannot get rid of HIV and cure a person of HIV disease. HIV becomes part of a person's body; there is no way yet to completely remove the virus. This means that medicines have to be taken for life. This leads to another problem: if a person does take medicines against HIV regularly, the medicines eventually stop working because the virus gets used to them. Furthermore, even though they fight HIV, these drugs sometimes harm the person who takes them.

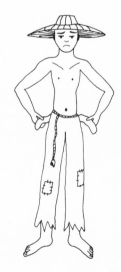

Drugs that work against HIV are sold at prices that are too expensive for most people.

Drugs for HIV are expensive, however activists have fought to make drug companies lower their prices for people living in poor countries. Currently the drugs usually cost between $250 and $750 per year. Many governments and organizations are also providing these drugs for free either through their own funding or with the support of international donors. Poor countries are also now making or buying generic versions of these drugs, so they are becoming more available.

The future

People are trying to make a vaccine to prevent HIV. Vaccines protect people against infections by causing the body to make antibodies. Vaccines help the immune system remember how a virus "looks"; the next time the immune system sees the virus, it attacks quickly, before a person becomes sick. For example, if someone has been vaccinated against mumps, his body makes antibodies, just as if he had a real infection with mumps. People do not get mumps twice. So, people who have been vaccinated against mumps do not get the disease. This is the way vaccines prevent infection. It will take many years to develop a good vaccine for HIV, so changing people's behavior is, for now, the only method to stop the spread of the virus.

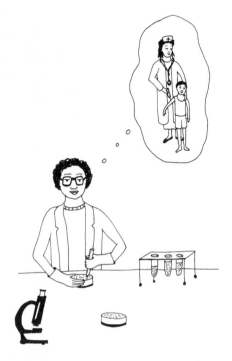

It will take many years to develop a good vaccine against HIV.

Answering Shoba's questions

"What is HIV? How does HIV cause AIDS? Why can't the body overcome AIDS like it can the flu? Are there pills to cure AIDS?"

HIV is neither an animal nor a plant. It is a virus. A virus lives inside plants, animals, or fungi and uses these (its "hosts") to survive. Diseases caused by viruses include the flu, chicken pox, mumps, polio, and herpes, as well as

AIDS. It is especially difficult for the body's defenses to fight HIV because it hides in the cells of the immune system—the very cells that are used to defend the body. The weakened immune system is unable to fight off infections that are usually not a problem for healthy people. In this way HIV causes AIDS, a group of diseases that occur when HIV has damaged a person's immune system. HIV is so damaging to the immune system that without treatment, most people with HIV will die from AIDS. This is why it is so important to teach people how to avoid getting or spreading HIV, and to strengthen their immune systems by fighting malnutrition and other diseases.

There is no medicine that can cure AIDS or even rid a person of HIV. But medicines can reduce the amount of HIV in a person's body and can treat the illnesses or opportunistic infections that affect people with HIV. These medicines can help people with HIV to live much longer, healthier lives. People with HIV can also stay healthier when they have clean water to drink, good nutrition, and support from their communities.

2

The symptoms of HIV infection

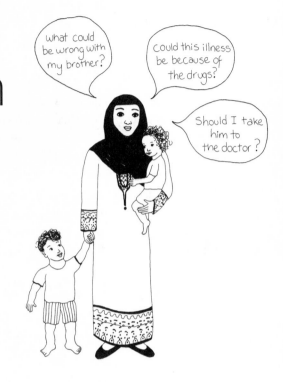

Saleema's story

HIV infection and HIV disease

The first weeks of HIV infection

The quiet stage of HIV infection

The beginning of HIV disease

Answering Saleema's questions

Saleema's story

Saleema is a young mother in a small village in Morocco. She has two children. Her husband works in the nearby fields. Saleema's parents both died when she was very young. When they died her brother, Hamid, moved to Paris, France, to look for work. An uncle there helped him get a job as a taxi driver. It was hard work but Hamid was able to send some money to help Saleema and her sisters. After some time Hamid became tired of his life in the city and returned to the village to work in the fields. Saleema was glad to see him but could not believe how he had changed. He was thin and felt very tired all the time. She wonders what could be wrong with him. He has fevers and sweats at night, and he seems to always have a cough and diarrhea that no medicine will cure. Saleema wants to take him to the doctor. Hamid told her that while in Paris he used drugs to try to take away his loneliness. She asks you, "What could be wrong with Hamid? Why does he have sweats at night and swollen lumps in his armpits and neck? Could this illness be because of the drugs? Should I take him to the doctor?"

HIV infection and HIV disease

HIV damages many parts of a person's body. It can do this in two ways: one is by directly invading different organs, the other is by weakening the immune system and allowing other organisms to cause disease. In this chapter we will describe the first kind of damage that HIV causes; in the Appendix we discuss the second.

HIV directly infects the cells in a person's brain, nervous system, intestines, and blood. HIV damages these cells. This affects the way a person thinks (from damage to the brain), causes pain or numbness in arms and legs (from damage to the nerves), causes diarrhea (from damage to the intestines), and causes anemia and bleeding (from damage to the blood). Although HIV can cause people to be ill, we already know that not everyone with HIV is sick. This is because there are different stages to HIV infection, beginning with the time when a person is first infected, moving through a period when no symptoms are present, reaching a time when symptoms first appear, and ending with advanced HIV disease (AIDS).

The four stages of HIV infection

1. The first few weeks after infection, when many people have symptoms like the flu.
2. The quiet period, when there are few signs of HIV disease.
3. Early HIV disease.
4. Advanced HIV disease (AIDS), when a person is very ill.

Over time, one stage leads to the next.

The first weeks of HIV infection

The first stage of HIV infection occurs after a person is infected with the virus. Usually people do not notice when they get HIV; they do not find out that they have the virus until later, when they are tested or become ill. A few people, however, do notice symptoms 1–4 weeks after they are infected with the virus. The symptoms are much like the symptoms of the flu: sore throat, fever, headache, stomach pain, diarrhea, and a feeling of being tired. After a week, a rash may appear on the chest, face, and neck. People may also have night sweats, muscle and joint pains, swelling in their lymph nodes, nausea, and vomiting. These symptoms usually last fewer than two weeks.

Rarely, the first stage of HIV infection can be more serious and damage a person's nervous system. The infected person may develop swelling of the brain and its covering. This can cause headache, neck stiffness, fever, confusion, nervous system problems, and coma. A person may also have problems with the nerves in the arms and legs, and problems with nerves in the face. This can cause pain, numbness, or difficulty moving. The lymph nodes can sometimes swell and stay swollen for months or even years.

Because all of these symptoms are also seen in illnesses other than HIV, we cannot say that a person has HIV just because he has one or more of these symptoms. For a person to know whether he has HIV, he needs to be tested for the virus. Unfortunately, HIV tests do not work well in the first few weeks after infection, because the tests look for antibodies, and the body of someone who has just become infected with HIV has not made antibodies yet. Most people will have antibodies within three weeks of getting HIV. Someone who thinks she may have just been infected with HIV can get tested right away and again a few weeks later. (For more about HIV testing, see Chapters 7 and 8.)

Lymph nodes

Lymph nodes, often called "glands," are the centers of a person's immune system. They become swollen and painful when a person is fighting off an infection. For example, lymph nodes in the neck often swell when a person has a throat infection. HIV also causes swollen lymph nodes, sometimes all over a person's body, and sometimes for years.

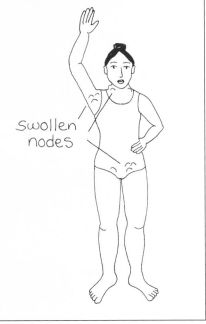

Swollen nodes

The quiet stage of HIV infection

People recover from the first symptoms of HIV infection within a few days or weeks. For several years after that they feel well, look healthy, and carry on with their daily lives. Their immune systems are able to fight the virus.

This is called the "incubation period," or the quiet stage of HIV. It is the time between the first infection with HIV and the point where a person becomes ill from the virus. For adults, this stage averages ten years. Right now, most of the people in the world who have HIV are in this incuba-

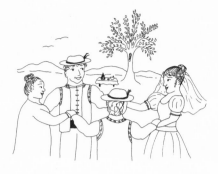

tion period. They are not experiencing any symptoms, and many of them do not even know they have the virus and could spread it.

The beginning of HIV disease

After the incubation period, people with HIV become ill. The virus weakens their immune systems enough that they develop infections that people with healthy immune systems are able to fight off. These infections—called "opportunistic infections"—and some cancers are what make people with HIV ill and define their illness as AIDS. We discuss treatments for them in the appendix. At the same time that their immune systems are weakening, people with HIV often develop swollen lymph nodes and lose weight. These general symptoms are common in people with HIV and are often not due to any specific infection.

HIV, weight loss, and malnutrition

Many people live in communities where food is scarce and where malnutrition is a serious problem. Not only do people need enough food, they need different kinds of food. For example, a person who is eating cassava and nothing else will become very ill. If a person is sick from not getting enough of the right kinds of food, he has malnutrition. Malnutrition can cause diseases as well as weight loss. One of the most important ways of staying healthy is to eat well and drink clean water. This is especially true for people with HIV and AIDS. They are likely to become malnourished from constantly being sick, from diarrhea that prevents their bodies from absorbing the nutrients in food, from loss of appetite, and from mouth infections that make eating difficult. Weight loss is so common in people with HIV that in some areas of Africa AIDS is called "slim disease."

Eating a balanced diet of different foods helps people with HIV stay strong and healthy. A balanced diet is one in which different foods from all of the basic nutrient groups are eaten each day. The basic nutrients are proteins, carbohydrates, fats and oils, and vitamins and minerals.

The basic nutrient groups

Proteins help the body grow and heal. Foods that have high amounts of protein include fish and other seafood, meat (for example, beef, pork, lamb, and goat), fowl (for example, chicken, turkey, and duck), eggs, milk, cheese, beans, rice, peas, cereals, nuts, tofu, and other soybean products.

Carbohydrates give the body energy. Starches and sugars are types of carbohydrates. Starches are in corn, rice, wheat, oats, buckwheat, millet, noodles, plain and sweet potatoes, squash, cassava, plantains, and taro. Sugars are found in sugarcane, beets, refined sugar, candy, honey, and fruit. Starches in potatoes and wheat give the body a steady source of energy. Refined sugars such as candy give the body sugar and no other nutrients. Eating too many sugars can also cause tooth decay and gum disease.

Fats and oils help the body store energy. There is twice as much energy in fat as in protein or carbohydrates. This means that eating fats and oils helps people gain weight. Fats and oils also taste good. The problem with fat for many people is that it causes them to have heart disease and to be overweight. This is usually not a problem for people with HIV, because they are trying to gain weight. Foods with fat include oil, lard, butter, margarine, nuts, sesame, soybean, coconut, avocado, cream, milk, and red meat like beef, pork, and lamb.

Vitamins and minerals are necessary in small amounts for a person's health. They are contained in many different foods, especially vegetables and fruits. This is one reason a varied diet is important for a person's health—it gives a variety of vitamins and minerals.

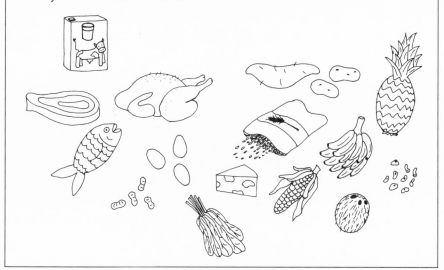

If someone has trouble eating

People with HIV may have nausea and vomiting. Teas or medicines may help with this. For people with mouth sores, cool, non-spicy foods make eating less painful. For people who have trouble swallowing, moving the head forward and using softer foods will make swallowing easier. Care should be taken when drinking to avoid choking. Drinking through a straw may help. Sometimes problems with eating or swallowing may be due to a disease that can be treated, like a yeast infection in the mouth. In these cases, encourage people to see a health worker for treatment.

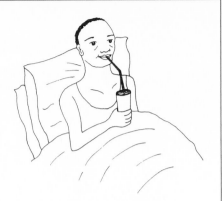

Women and children have special nutritional needs. This is because women lose a lot of nutrients through menses, pregnancy, and breast-feeding. Children need extra food because they are growing quickly. Women and children who have HIV need even more food to stay healthy because HIV places more demands on their bodies.

In HIV disease, each infection needs to be treated as well as possible. The Appendix discusses treatments for the most common diseases that affect people with HIV.

Answering Saleema's questions

"What could be wrong with Hamid? Why does he have sweats at night and swollen lumps in his armpits and neck? Could this illness be because of the drugs? Should I take him to the doctor?"

Hamid is very sick and needs to see a doctor to find out what is wrong. The fact that he used drugs while in Paris means he is at high risk for HIV disease, especially if he injected them. People with HIV usually do not know when they got the virus because the first symptoms are like having a bad cold. Later, people have swollen lymph nodes, night sweats, and diarrhea. Hamid has all of these symptoms, and he has lost weight. These are bad signs. If he has HIV, there are medicines that can help him. If Hamid does not have HIV but another disease, like tuberculosis, then he will also need treatment. It is important to find out so that Hamid can get help.

3

Who has HIV?

Min-Soo's story

Min-Soo is a student in your health training class. He comes from a village on the edge of a large town in South Korea. Recently a person in his community was diagnosed with AIDS. People are scared. Min-Soo is working with a project that teaches people about HIV. His friends have asked him many questions. They have asked where AIDS came from and which country has the most AIDS. They also want to know who gets HIV. Min-Soo knows these questions are about the "epidemiology" of HIV. He stays after your lesson to ask some more questions. "Where was AIDS first found? Which country has the most AIDS? How do we know that HIV is not spread by mosquitoes or sneezing? What does it really mean when they say that 15% of adults living in the capital of Rwanda have HIV?"

A short history of the HIV epidemic

HIV and AIDS have spread to almost all countries in the world. The virus is so common now that in some communities one of every 3 or 4 young adults are infected. When a disease becomes this widespread, it is called an epidemic. Epidemiology is the study of diseases in populations. It can be used to understand the spread of HIV. We must understand the spread of HIV if we are to stop the epidemic.

The first official case of AIDS was found in 1981 in the United States, but researchers believe that by that time many people all over the world had HIV. They think that in 1980, about 100,000 people worldwide had HIV. Most of the people who had the virus were not sick and did not realize they were infected. Today, over 39 million people, including 2 million children, have HIV. This is almost 400 times the number of people infected in 1980. You can see that HIV is spreading quickly to people all over the world.

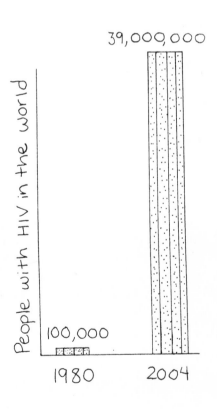

The number of people with HIV in the world is growing.

HIV in the world

Over 39 million people with HIV

around 22 million men

around 17 million women

Of the 39 million

around 80% got HIV during sex; of these, 80% got HIV during sex between men and women

around 10% got HIV during injection drug use

around 5% are children infected by mothers who have HIV

around 5% got HIV through blood

Numbers of people with HIV in different parts of the world

around 26 million in Africa

around 1 million in North America

around 2 million in Latin America

around 8 million in Asia

around 2 million in Europe and Central Asia

Because HIV is spreading so quickly, we cannot know exactly how many people have it. The HIV epidemic is like a fire that is spreading through a forest—by the time you have put out part of it, you find it has moved to a new area of the woods.

Global cooperation

Sometimes HIV seems like some other country's or community's problem. It is easy to find another community that has more infections than yours. But because we are all connected, HIV is a threat to everyone. A global view is needed to stop the spread of HIV.

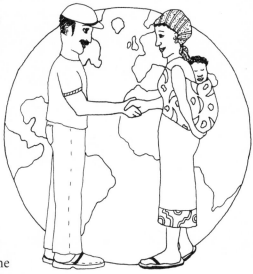

In the beginning of the AIDS epidemic, people pointed fingers at other people or countries and blamed them for the problem. This happens with almost every new disease. Some people in the United States said HIV came from Africa and the Caribbean and that homosexual men (men who have sex only with men) were the cause. Now we know that this is not true, but countries in Africa and the Caribbean were insulted by the finger-pointing.

In the past, some countries were afraid to admit that they had people with AIDS for fear of losing money from tourists. Some of these countries are now openly saying that HIV is a problem for them. They are working with the international community to stop AIDS. Understanding that HIV and AIDS are a problem for every country and taking action to stop its spread are important for the world. Countries that ignored the epidemic have more HIV and AIDS now than many of those that worked toward stopping the spread of the virus early. In the end, it is not important to know where the virus started. It *is* important to know where it is going.

How HIV is spread worldwide

More than 300 million people cross international boundaries each year. Changes in transportation have made it easier for HIV to spread. Someone with the virus can travel from London, England to a small village in Asia in a day. If he has unsafe sex with a person in the village, HIV can spread across the world with him. The same can occur if someone from a village visits a city, becomes infected, and returns home. This is how the virus moves. It spreads from person to person, village to village, and city to city. For a virus like HIV there are no borders. Where people move, HIV moves.

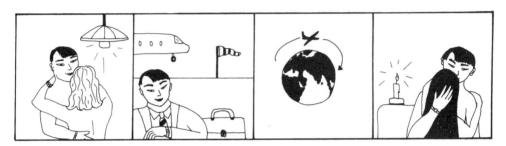

As we said in Chapter 1, HIV can only be spread through sex, blood, dirty needles or other instruments, and from a mother to her baby. HIV does not necessarily affect the same people first in every community. For example, in India most people with HIV got the virus from having heterosexual sex—sex between a man and a woman. In Russia most people with HIV got the virus from sharing used needles while injecting drugs. There are a few reasons why people who take part in a particular risky behavior may be affected first or affected more by HIV:

Cities and disease

Half of the world's population lives in cities. Diseases like tuberculosis and the flu spread more quickly in the city because people are crowded together. HIV also spreads faster in cities, for many reasons. For example, people in cities tend to have sex with a greater number of partners. More people move to cities every year. As more people move to cities it is likely that HIV will spread even faster than it already does.

- Certain behaviors (like injecting drugs) may be more common in some countries or regions.
- The first people to contract HIV in a certain region will pass the virus on within their own communities. So if a gay man (a man who only has sex with other men) is the first to be infected in a certain town, he will pass the virus on to other men who have sex with men in that town first.

Because a certain group of people may be the first to get HIV, others in the community may see HIV as only affecting people who are members of that group. But unless the whole community works to stop HIV right away, it will quickly spread and infect people from many different parts of the community. HIV may be seen as a disease of gay men, or of drug users, of prostitutes, or of unfaithful husbands. But HIV will infect anyone who is exposed, including faithful wives, newborn babies, and people who have never taken illegal drugs.

Effects of HIV on the community

Most people with HIV are adults from 20 to 40 years of age. This means people are dying at an age when they are vital members of their communities. Illness and death at these ages affect the strength and productivity of a community. In most places, women and men between the ages of 20 and 40 take care of their own children and sometimes even their parents, grandparents, or grandchildren. When these men and women die, children and the elderly are often left without support. AIDS has killed either one or both parents of millions of children around the world. In most countries there are not enough orphanages to support all of the children whose parents die from AIDS. This is just one way AIDS changes families and communities.

The spread of HIV has also changed health care. More hospital beds are needed for people who are sick with AIDS. Because hospitals and clinics are so busy, less attention can be given to everyone who is sick. In one African country, three top officials of the ministry of health died of AIDS in one year. There was no one in the country who was qualified to replace them. This affected the health of the entire country.

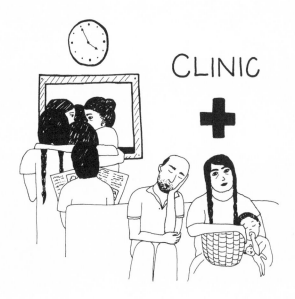

Because of HIV, hospitals and clinics have become even more crowded.

War and HIV

War can increase the spread of HIV in many ways. During wartime soldiers move from place to place. Soldiers with HIV or other sexually transmitted diseases spread them to new communities.

Soldiers also often attack clinics and hospitals. This means that services such as HIV counseling, testing, and medical care may stop. Sometimes hospitals and clinics are forced to close.

During war, parents are killed and families broken apart. Because men in particular may be killed or sent away to fight, the meaning of social customs such as marriage and sex also changes. Husbands and wives may have more sex partners when they are separated.

As people lose their homes and animals, fear and hunger make them leave the countryside for the protection of cities. War often brings poverty and despair, driving people into drug use or prostitution. These changes make it easier for HIV to spread to people who before might have been safe from the virus.

War changes people's ideas about life. When people are surrounded by so much upheaval and death, they do not worry about catching HIV because it does not kill for years, whereas bullets or bombs may kill them tomorrow.

In the late 1970s, a war occurred in southern and western Uganda. This war made it easier for HIV to spread. It left many people homeless, poor, or living as refugees in the capital. With the movement of troops, the arrival of truck drivers from the coast, and the new refugees, HIV spread rapidly. By the mid-1990s, 10% to 25% of the younger people in some areas of Uganda had HIV, and over a million children were orphaned by HIV.

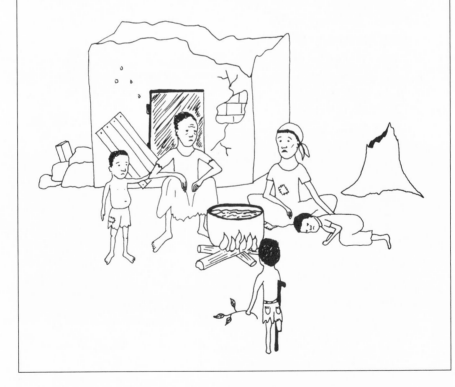

HIV and other diseases

People with HIV are more likely than people without HIV to get certain cancers like Kaposi's sarcoma and lymphoma, and opportunistic infections like cryptococcal meningitis and thrush. Some people have worried that these diseases would spread to people without HIV. But these cancers and infections do not spread to other people. So far the only disease that people with HIV are likely to spread to other people is tuberculosis (TB).

The epidemiology of tuberculosis and HIV

People with HIV live many years before they become ill. People infected with tuberculosis (TB) can also live many years without becoming ill, because the bacteria that cause TB can live quietly in a person. Unfortunately, people who have HIV and TB infection become ill with TB much more often than people who do not have HIV.

$$500,000 \times 50\% = 250,000 \text{ with TB}$$

Most of the diseases that people with HIV get are not passed to others. TB is different in that it can be spread to other people. About 5% of people with HIV and TB infection will become sick from TB each year. It is believed that in some areas of the world, around 50% of the people are already infected with TB. The spread of HIV is especially dangerous for these people.

$$250,000 \times 25\% = 62,500 \text{ with TB and HIV}$$

Find a pencil and paper and follow the numbers in this imaginary example:

The town of Mycolandia in East Africa has 500,000 people and 50% of them are infected with TB. This means that 250,000 people have TB in their body. Most are not sick from TB. The TB bacteria are just living quietly.

$$62,500 \times 5\% = 3,125 \text{ with HIV who become ill with TB every year}$$

In Mycolandia, 25% of the people have HIV. This means 25% of the 250,000 people infected with TB also have HIV. In other words, 62,500 people have both infections.

If 5% of people with both TB and HIV infection become sick with tuberculosis in one year, that means that 3,125 people with HIV will become ill with TB disease each year. Each person who becomes ill with TB can spread it to other people. If a person with TB is treated with the right antibiotics, he will no longer spread the TB bacteria and he will feel better.

How do we study the HIV epidemic?

The HIV epidemic can be divided into two parts: people with HIV and people with AIDS. People with HIV who do not have AIDS are difficult to count because they usually are not ill. You need a test to know if someone has HIV. It is easier to count how many people have AIDS because they are sick from HIV disease and usually go to a health worker for treatment. The World Health Organization (WHO) has a definition of AIDS that uses the presence of certain diseases and does not require a blood test (see the first box in the appendix, and the second and third boxes from the end of the appendix). It takes many years for people with HIV to get AIDS. If we only count people with AIDS, we will think that many fewer people have HIV than really do.

It is too expensive to test everyone for HIV. This is where the tools of epidemiology, such as screening (testing groups of people) and surveillance (regularly monitoring the rates of a disease), come in handy. By testing certain groups of people and using math, it is possible to come up with an idea of how many people have HIV, who they are, and where they are living.

Let us imagine you want to know how many women giving birth in your city have HIV. One way is to test every woman giving birth. But this would cost too much if you live in a big city where many women give birth each year. Another way would be to choose two or three hospitals from different parts of the city and spend one month testing every woman giving birth. The results of this study could be used to get a general idea of how many women giving birth in the city have HIV. If 500 women gave birth at the hospitals where you did testing and 50 had HIV, then 10% of all women giving birth at the hospitals in a one-month period had HIV. If you already know that in the entire city, about 1,000 women give birth to babies in a one-month period, then you could multiply 10% by 1,000 and estimate that about 100 women with HIV give birth to children every month in the city. This means that in a year, about 1,200 women with HIV give birth to children in the city. This number is an estimate.

An estimate is a best guess. Sometimes estimates are not correct. You can get an idea of how good an estimate is by thinking about where your calculations might be wrong. For example, if the hospitals where you did your testing were in parts of the city where many people with HIV live, then the number of women with HIV giving birth would be higher there than in other hospitals in the city. This would mean 1,200 is an overestimate and the true number is less. Good estimates provide information that can be used to focus resources without having to test everyone, but be careful: bad estimates can lead to bad decisions and wasted resources.

In New York City in the United States, studies of drug injectors showed that sharing needles spread HIV. Around 70% of the people injecting illegal drugs had HIV. Less than 1% of the rest of the population had HIV. Studies like this one helped people plan special programs to try to stop the spread of HIV among drug injectors. If in your community only a small percentage of drug injectors have HIV, then it would be espe-

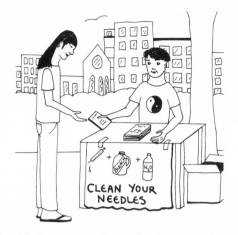

cially useful to set up a program to talk with drug users about the dangers of sharing used needles, to show them how to sterilize needles, and, if possible, to provide them with new, clean needles. This could keep the rate of HIV infection low. Do not wait until most drug injectors are already infected to start your work.

Question the experts and their studies

How do we know the number of people with HIV in a country? It would be very difficult to test all of the people living in any country. Instead, people test different groups and estimate what percentage of the entire population is infected. When someone says that 10% of people in an area have HIV, a few questions should come to mind. The first question to ask is, "Who is saying this?" Is it someone who is actually testing people and who would know about how many people are positive, or is it someone who is just guessing? Ask how the study was done. Who was tested? Was it only people in a big city? If so, the estimated number is likely to be higher than the true number for the whole region, because in most parts of the world, people in cities are more likely to have HIV. Were only sex workers tested? If so, the estimate will be higher than the true number in the general population, because sex workers are more likely to have HIV. Were the people who were tested over 60 years old? If so, the estimate is likely to be lower than it should be, because people over 60 are less likely to have HIV than people in their twenties. Most of epidemiology is based on estimates, so be careful and ask questions!

Epidemiology can also be used to find out what happens to people once they have HIV. Questions such as "How long do people with AIDS live? With what diseases do people with HIV become sick? How do they die? What medicines help?" can be answered by closely watching people with HIV and carrying out studies.

The words that people use to talk about the spread of disease can be confusing. Here are some definitions:

Rate. Rate is one of the most important ideas in epidemiology. Rate is the amount of something in relation to something else. It is usually shown as a proportion or percentage. Often it contains the idea of time. For example, imagine that 10,000 cases of AIDS have been reported to the ministry of health over the past ten years. You could tell someone this information alone, or you could say that the country only has a population of 100,000 people, and the rate of AIDS is 0.1, or 10% (10,000 cases divided by 100,000 people).

Ten thousand cases is more serious in this country than in a country where 10,000,000 people live. In the second country, the rate of AIDS is 0.001, or 0.1% (10,000 cases divided by 10,000,000 people). You can see how the number of cases of AIDS or HIV infection is often less important than the rate of disease or infection. When someone tells you the number of people with AIDS in an area, always ask for the number of people living there. This will give you an idea of the rate of disease.

Incidence. The incidence of a disease is how often new cases of it appear in a population during a set period of time, usually one year. For example, if you wanted to know the incidence of HIV in a village, you could test all the people in the village and record that information as your baseline. Then test all of the same people one year later. Count the number of people who did not have HIV during the first test but did have the virus during the second test. Divide this number by the total number of uninfected people in the village. The result is the incidence of HIV in this village (the number of new infections per person per year).

Imagine that 1,000 people live in the village. One hundred of them had HIV the first time you tested them. One year later, 150 people had HIV. This means 50 new people were infected. Fifty new infections among the 900 people who were not originally infected means the incidence of HIV infections was 0.055, or 5.5%.

Prevalence. Prevalence is the proportion of people who have a disease in a community at any one point in time. In the example above, the prevalence of HIV would be 10% the first year (100 cases among 1,000 people living in the village) and 15% the second year (150 cases among 1,000 people living in the village).

Bias. Bias occurs when an unexpected factor affects the results of a study. For example, imagine you want to find out how many pregnant women in your town have HIV. You test all the pregnant women who come to your medical clinic over a three-month period. Since people with HIV are more likely to be sick and come to the clinic, and you tested all pregnant women who came to the clinic, you will find more women with HIV than if you tested every pregnant woman in the town. Testing only sick pregnant women influenced your results. Your study was affected by bias. Bias can happen even when you are trying to avoid it. If you ask questions with a tone that tells people that you want them to answer in a certain way, you can bias your results. For example, if you want to know how many people inject drugs but ask, "You do not use those illegal, deadly drugs do you?" then fewer people will answer yes than really do use drugs. Your results will be biased.

AIDS can be seen as the footprints that HIV has left as it spreads from person to person. Epidemiology is used to examine these footprints in order to understand where the virus is going and how to stop its spread. Knowing the size of the HIV problem in your community helps you prepare for the future. Education and prevention programs can involve the people who need them most. By continuing to gather information about HIV you will know whether or not you are slowing the spread of HIV.

Answering Min-Soo's questions

"Where was AIDS first found? Which country has the most AIDS? How do we know that HIV is not spread by mosquitoes or sneezing? What does it really mean when they say that 15% of adults living in the capital of Rwanda have HIV?"

AIDS was first described in 1981 in Los Angeles in the United States, when five patients became sick with an unusual pneumonia that occurred in people with weak immune systems. The virus causing AIDS was found by a group in France a few years later.

From studying the epidemiology of AIDS, we know that HIV is not spread by mosquitoes or sneezing. Almost all people with HIV can trace their infection back to sex, blood, dirty needles or instruments, or from mother to baby at birth. If mosquitoes could spread HIV, then AIDS would be seen in the same people who have malaria. We would see more children and old people with HIV. This is not the case. Similarly, HIV is not spread through sneezing or other "casual contact" with people who have HIV. Health care workers do not get the virus through casual contact, even though they spend many hours caring for people who have HIV. Within families, HIV is spread only through sex or from a mother to her baby; people do not get ill from living with and caring for family members who have HIV.

No one has tested all of the adults living in the capital of Rwanda for HIV. What people have done is tested a group of people and estimated what percentage of the entire population is infected. Thus, 15% is a statistical guess. You can explain to Min-Soo that the idea that 15% of the adults in the capital of Rwanda have HIV is an estimate made from several different studies.

4

HIV around the world

Is it too dangerous to study in the United States?

Isn't it true that people are dying in the street from AIDS?

Lon Chin's story

Lon Chin is a student in a small town near Xian in central China, where her parents raise ducks. She worked very hard in high school and was chosen to go to the national university in Beijing. She did very well at the university and was the top student in her English class. During her last year she won a scholarship to study English in the United States. She was very excited, but her parents were afraid to let her go. "It is too dangerous to study in the United States. Isn't it true that people are dying in the streets from AIDS? Besides, we don't want you to live in dormitories with students from Africa, India, and Latin America, where AIDS is so common." Lon Chin became frightened herself.

Not knowing what was true, she decided to ask you, her local health worker, for answers.

HIV in different regions of the world

Each day about 15,000 people are newly infected with HIV. Who is infected, and how they got HIV, is different in different areas of the world. When HIV first appears in a country, most infections occur in people who frequently have unsafe sex, especially with more than one partner; in people who inject drugs; or in people who have had blood transfusions. These people make up a small percentage of the whole population, but they are at high risk of infection. This is the early stage of the epidemic. North America is in this stage; there, most HIV infections have occurred among drug injectors, their sexual partners, and men who have sex with men.

However, over time, infections spread to others. Sometimes this happens very quickly. For example, in Africa south of the Sahara Desert, HIV quickly spread among sex workers, through transfusions of HIV-infected blood, and along truck routes, where truck drivers and travelers spread the infection from community to community. Now, most people newly infected with HIV are under the age of 25, most are infected through sexual contact between women and men, and many are married. The rate of HIV infection is high, and in many cities over 30% of adults have HIV. Babies are often infected with HIV. This pattern is most common in countries where HIV has been present for a long time. There, the HIV epidemic is at a late stage.

In both the late and early stages of an HIV epidemic, much can be done to prevent new infections. In fact, in several countries the news is good. In Uganda, a country with a late-stage epidemic, the number of people newly infected with HIV has dropped because volunteers, health workers, and the government have run prevention programs and educated the public. In Thailand, another country with a late-stage epidemic, a "100% condom use" campaign promoting condom use among sex workers has lowered the number of new infections among young men in the army. In the United States, the number of drug injectors newly infected with HIV has dropped in certain cities because of education and needle-exchange programs (see Chapter 12).

In 2004, almost 5 million people were newly infected with HIV; 640,000 of these were children. Most of these people live in the less industrialized countries of the world. Most people with HIV in the world today do not even know that they have the virus.

Information used in this chapter was collected by the United Nations AIDS program (UNAIDS). Most of the numbers are estimates of the true number of cases of HIV or AIDS. For cases of AIDS, the numbers are *reported* cases, not the true number of cases, because some countries have more money, more HIV testing, and better reporting than other countries. Some countries are able to report a higher number of cases not because they really have more, but because they have had more reported. Also, a few countries do not want others to know how much HIV they have and do not report all of their AIDS cases. No country can diagnose and report every case of AIDS, but some do better than others. The total number of people with HIV or AIDS is often not as important as the percentage of people infected (see Chapter 3). A country with a small population and 10,000 cases of AIDS has a much more serious problem than a country with a large population and the same number of cases.

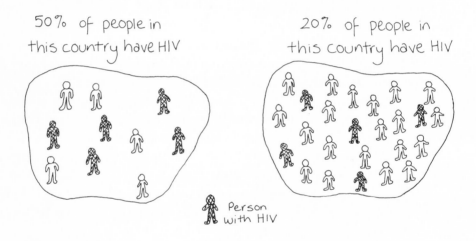

Both countries have the same number of people with HIV, but the country with the smaller population has a more serious HIV problem—50% of the people living there have HIV.

Men, women, and HIV

In most countries in Africa, the number of women who have HIV is equal to or greater than the number of men with HIV. This is because in Africa the virus is mainly spread through sex between women and men. In some other countries more men have HIV than women. This is true in the United States, where HIV spread very quickly among drug injectors and men who have sex

People living with HIV

Region	Adults & children living with HIV	Adult prevalence rate
Africa South of the Sahara	25,400,000	7.4%
South & Southeast Asia	7,100,000	0.6%
Latin America	1,700,000	0.6%
Eastern Europe & Central Asia	1,400,000	0.8%
East Asia & Pacific	1,100,000	0.1%
North America	1,000,000	0.6%
Western Europe	610,000	0.3%
North Africa & Middle East	540,000	0.3%
Caribbean	440,000	2.3%
Australia & New Zealand	35,000	0.2%
	39,325,000 total	1.1% worldwide average

with men. However, the ratio of men to women with HIV is changing in the United States because men who have sex with men are more often having "safer sex" (see Chapter 5), and the virus has continued to spread to women through sex and drug use. In a few years we expect the number of women newly infected with HIV to be greater than the number of men.

Women and HIV	
Region	Percentage of adults living with HIV who are women
Africa South of the Sahara	57%
North Africa & Middle East	48%
South & Southeast Asia	30%
Eastern Europe & Central Asia	34%
East Asia & Pacific	22%
Australia & New Zealand	21%
Western Europe	25%
North America	25%
Latin America	36%
Caribbean	49%
	47% worldwide average

Africa South of the Sahara Desert

Most people with HIV live in Africa, in countries south of the Sahara Desert. Only 10% of the world's people live in this region, but 60% of people with HIV in the world live there. That is about 25.4 million people with HIV.

A commitment on the part of local activists and health workers and national and international governments has decreased the numbers of people getting HIV in a few places — the percentage of Ugandans with HIV has been decreasing for several years. But in other places, the rate just keeps going up. In South Africa, almost 30% of pregnant women had HIV in 2003. Because of HIV, the average age of death in Zimbabwe is only 34 years old, while in 1990 a Zimbabwean would have been expected to live to around 52.

The crisis of HIV in Africa has been particularly devastating to women. About 13 women become infected for every 10 men there.

HIV once mostly infected people living in cities or near main highways. Now it has spread to villages throughout most countries.

Latin America and the Caribbean

When HIV first appeared in Latin America in the 1980s, it mostly spread among drug injectors and men who had sex with men. Now nearly 2 million people in this region are living with HIV. There were 240,000 new HIV infections in 2004. During the same year there were 95,000 deaths due to AIDS. In Mexico as many as 15% of men who have sex with men are living with HIV. In the Dominican Republic 2% of adults have HIV. In Jamaica, girls are over 2.5 times as likely to have HIV as boys, because older, HIV infected men seek young girls to have sex with. Haiti's life expectancy is nearly 6 years less than it would be if there was no AIDS epidemic. Brazil's success in giving antiretroviral treatment to 105,000 people has avoided 234,000 hospitalizations and saved many lives between 1996 and 2000. Despite increased treatment for AIDS, in Latin America and the Caribbean AIDS kills more people each year than traffic accidents.

North America and Western Europe

In North America and Western Europe, HIV first spread between men having sex with each other and also drug users sharing needles. Now HIV has spread into all social groups and is frequently spread by sex between men and women. In Western Europe in 1997, 25% of new HIV diagnoses were of women. In 2002, women accounted for 38% of new cases.

While rates of HIV are still slowly increasing in the US, deaths from AIDS have gone down since antiretroviral drugs became available there in 1995. Most people with HIV in the wealthy countries of North America and Western Europe have reliable access to these medicines.

As in most of the world, HIV has the worst effect on people who are poor and who experience other kinds of discrimination. In the US, where 1 of every 4 African Americans lives in poverty, the rate of HIV is disproportionately high in that group. 12% of people in the US are African American, but 25% of people with HIV are African American. Among new cases of HIV in women, 72% are found in African Americans.

Just like in many other areas of the world, HIV is more common in cities than in rural areas. In many large cities, including New York City, AIDS has become the number one cause of death in adults between 20 and 40 years of age. By the end of 2000, New York City had reported 118,123 cases of AIDS.

South and Southeast Asia

HIV started to spread in South and Southeast Asia in the early 1990s. This is later than in other areas of the world, but the number of people infected has increased very rapidly. Over 1 million people were infected with HIV in 2004 and there are now over 8 million people in South and Southeast Asia living with HIV. Currently, more than 5 million people in India are living with HIV. The epidemic in China shows no sign of slowing down and new HIV infection rates are increasing. China has few programs to teach people about HIV prevention.

In Cambodia and Thailand where there are large prevention programs, new HIV cases are decreasing. In Thailand where people have learned to use condoms, HIV is spreading less through sex. There are few programs to help prevent HIV among drug users though, and 30% of drug injectors are infected.

Eastern Europe and Central Asia

In Eastern Europe, the HIV crisis is still in its early stage. More than 1 million people have HIV in this region. Over 80% of these infections are among people who are younger than 30 years old.

In the Russian Federation injecting illegal drugs such as heroin or methamphetamines is very common. As many as 2% of the people there use these drugs. Right now, most HIV cases in Russia are found among drug users. They can then pass the disease to others by sharing needles or through sex. In the Ukraine, 30% of new infections now occur during sex between a man and a woman.

Many changes are taking place in this part of the world including wars and changing of national borders. These conditions often hasten the spread of disease.

Answering Lon Chin's questions

"It is too dangerous to study in the United States. Isn't it true that people are dying in the streets from AIDS? Besides, we don't want you to live in dormitories with students from Africa, India, and Latin America, where AIDS is so common."

You can tell Lon Chin that many people in the United States have HIV and AIDS. But just like everywhere else in the world, HIV is only spread through unsafe sex, from a mother to her baby, through dirty needles and other instruments, and through transfusions of HIV-infected blood. The United States tests its blood supply for HIV, which means that the blood supply is safe. Although many people in the United States have HIV, they make up only a small percentage of the millions of people living in the country. Also, when people with AIDS die, they usually do so in a hospital or at home—not in the street.

Studying with people from Africa, India, and Latin America has never caused anyone to get HIV. HIV is not spread by studying! Many places in the world have an HIV problem. Only knowledge of how the virus is spread will help people avoid the virus. If Lon Chin does not have unsafe sex or use drugs, then she is as safe from HIV in the United States as she is in China—or anywhere else.

5

Counseling about sexual behavior

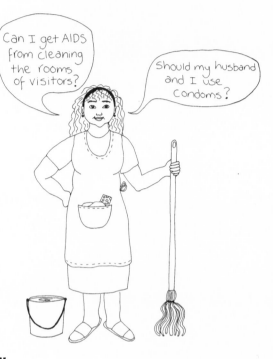

Olga's story

HIV and discrimination

Helping people change behavior

Casual contact and HIV

Sex and HIV

How to avoid spreading HIV through sex

Other factors that affect the spread of HIV

Answering Olga's questions

Olga's story

Olga works as a maid in a hotel in Tashkent, Uzbekistan. With her country's new independence, more foreigners have been traveling to Tashkent, and there has been news about several cases of AIDS. Because she cleans hotel rooms where foreigners stay, Olga has become worried. Most mornings she passes by your information table outside of the post office on her way to work. Today she stops and asks you, "Can I get AIDS from cleaning the rooms of German and American visitors? Should my husband and I use condoms to avoid giving each other AIDS?"

HIV and discrimination

People who do not understand how HIV is spread may discriminate against people with HIV—that is, they may treat them unfairly because they are afraid of getting the virus. Discrimination occurs not only against people with HIV but also against groups of people that are more likely to have HIV, such as sex workers, or are mistakenly thought to have HIV, such as foreigners. Teaching people about the real ways that HIV is spread protects them from the virus; teaching people about the ways that HIV is not spread protects everyone from unnecessary discrimination.

This chapter discusses how HIV can be spread during sex and how to have safer sex. The next chapter will discuss other ways that HIV can be transmitted.

Helping people change behavior

People can lower their chance of getting HIV by changing their behavior. The most important step in helping people change the way they act is to spark a desire to change. No one changes overnight. Small goals are often easier to reach than large ones. For example, never having sex is the surest way to avoid getting HIV through sex, but it is not realistic for most people. Stopping the use of drugs that are injected, like heroin, is another way to avoid HIV, but not everyone who uses drugs is able to stop. Taking small steps toward safer behavior will protect people more than no change at all. You may end up teaching people to use condoms until they and their partners can get tested, or to clean needles with bleach until they quit using drugs.

Sometimes a person does not have the choice to practice safer sex. Condoms may be too expensive to buy. A woman may not be able to ask her husband not to have other sexual partners. Take into account each person's life situation when you suggest ways to avoid HIV. Talking to people about how HIV is spread and how they can be safer will help them make their own decisions about their next step toward a safer lifestyle.

Changing behavior is hard work. There may be times when a person repeats unsafe practices. Do not give up; continue to encourage people to try to change unsafe behavior.

Casual contact and HIV

HIV is not spread by casual contact. The HIV virus cannot live in air, water, or food; it is weak and only lives in body fluids. It only spreads if the body fluid of a person with HIV gets inside another person. This is why shaking hands with people with HIV does not spread the virus. If this were *not* true, many more people would have HIV. Nurses, doctors, teachers, classmates, coworkers, friends, and family all touch people with HIV and do not get infected. People who live or work with people with HIV do not get the virus unless they have sex or share needles with them. The virus is not spread by doorknobs, typewriters, telephones, money, or anything else that has been touched by someone with HIV. HIV is not spread by hugging, touching, holding or shaking hands, dancing, using the toilet after someone with HIV, or eating food prepared by a person with HIV. People have shared dishes, towels, and bedsheets and still not become infected with HIV. No one has ever gotten HIV from sharing cigarettes, or being cried, sneezed, or spit on. Mosquitoes do not spread HIV. Other viruses like measles or chicken pox are spread easily through the air. We are lucky that HIV is so difficult to spread.

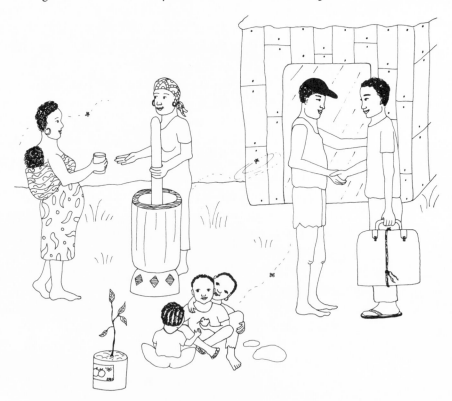

HIV is not spread by "casual" contact.

Sex and HIV

HIV *is* spread through sex. It can be spread from men to women and from women to men. It can also be spread among men and among women. A person can get HIV from a sexual partner who appears healthy but has HIV. Anyone can get HIV, not only sex workers and drug users—a judge, bartender, farmworker, or doctor can get HIV if she has sex with someone with the virus. It can infect people who are tall, fat, small, old, young, black, white, yellow, brown, male, female, mothers, fathers, brothers, and sisters. Anyone. Who a person is does not matter to the virus. What matters is what a person does. HIV does not discriminate by who you are, but by what you do.

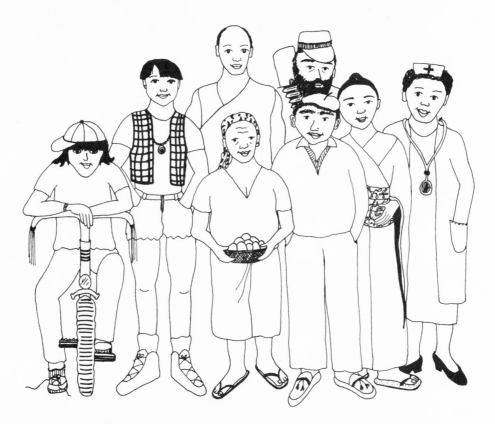

HIV does not discriminate by who you are.

A sure way to avoid getting HIV from sex is to never have sex. While having no sex is safe, most adults want to have sex. Knowing how HIV is spread, some people will choose never to have sex; others will choose to have sex only with one partner; and others will have several partners. Teaching people the risks involved will allow them to make choices that are based on fact.

Many people have sex but do not talk about it. Because of HIV and AIDS, this must change. Sexual partners have to talk about what they are doing. Talking about HIV before having sex is much better than talking about it afterward (or during!). Often people have thought about HIV but feel uncomfortable talking about it with their sexual partners. Those who finally talk about HIV usually feel relieved. This is especially true in places where anxiety about infection is common.

You can teach people how to talk about sex with their partners. One way is to have people role-play a discussion. Role playing works well because it takes an embarrassing and intimate situation and brings it into the open. It prepares people for the real thing (see Chapter 11).

One of the most important skills to teach people is how to say no. It can be difficult for people to say that they do not want to have sex. They may have trouble saying that they only want to kiss, or that they want to touch without having intercourse. It is common to feel awkward saying these things.

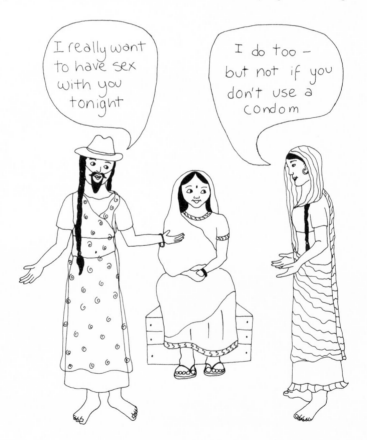

Role playing can be useful.

Refusal skills: How to say no

Here are some ways people in one country have said "no" when they did not want to have sex. You can use these or think of other ways that would work where you live.

Get the other person's attention:

Use his first name

Look into his eyes

Say "Listen to me"

Say no:

Use the words "I said no"

Use a firm voice

Hold your body in a way that says no

If pressured to have sex anyway:

Say no again

Suggest doing something else

Leave

Other ways to say no:

Use humor

Ask him why he cares so much about having sex; this puts the pressure on him

Keep repeating what you want

Tell your partner you need to think about it more

Questions to ask yourself:

Am I being pressured?

Do I need more information before I make a decision?

Is there a way I could avoid this situation in the future?

But everyone has the right to do only what she wants to do. Role playing can be useful for teaching people different ways to say no.

People often ask, "How can I have sex without getting HIV?" People with HIV do not always spread the virus during sex. Some people with HIV have had sex without condoms many times without giving their partners the virus. Some people with HIV have had sex only once and have given the virus to their partners. No one is sure exactly why this is true. Part of the reason is that the amount of virus in a person goes up and down over time. Another part of the reason is that some types of sexual acts have a higher chance of spreading HIV than others do. Understanding which types of sex have a higher chance

Understanding chance

When you toss a coin into the air, chances are it will fall on one side about half the time and on the other side half the time. Similarly, probability, or chance, tells us that about half the babies born in a town will be boys and the other half girls. What chance cannot say is whether a particular woman will have a boy or a girl.

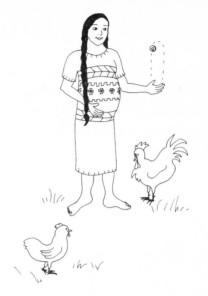

People take part in lotteries for money even when there is only a one in 100,000 chance that they will win the grand prize. Farmers buy calves and take a chance that they will be good milk producers when they grow up. Some people will not ride in an airplane or a car because they fear it will crash, even if there is very little chance this will happen. Every day we think about chance when we make decisions about our lives. What some people do not think about is that having sex has a chance of spreading HIV, just like buying a lottery ticket has a chance of leading to a prize. The difference is that one "rewards" with a deadly virus and the other rewards with money.

of spreading HIV helps people understand the risk they are taking. People can then talk with their partners about what kind of sex they want to have.

People use different words to talk about sex in different communities. It is helpful to learn and become comfortable using these words. Since this book cannot use all the words that people use locally, we will define and use only a few words. Some people use the words "vaginal sex" to discuss a woman having her vagina touched by her partner's mouth, fingers, penis, or other objects. We do not. We use the words "vaginal sex" only to talk about when a man's penis enters a woman's vagina. Similarly, we use the words "anal sex" only to describe when a man's penis enters a woman's or man's anus.

Sexual acts with no risk of spreading HIV

Some sexual acts have *never* spread HIV and are completely safe. People who have completely safe sex do not exchange body fluids such as semen, blood, vaginal fluid, or saliva. Safe sex is when only the outsides of people's bodies touch. This is safe even with people who are known to have HIV.

What kinds of sex risk spreading HIV?	
No risk	Low risk
Dry kissing	Wet kissing
Masturbation	Oral sex on a man or a woman
Touching, hugging, massage	Vaginal sex with a condom
Fantasizing	Anal sex with a condom
Rubbing bodies together	High risk
Kissing someone's body	Unprotected vaginal sex
	Unprotected anal sex

Safe sex includes using hands to touch a person's vagina, penis, anus, breasts, or nipples. It also includes "dry" kissing, hugging, or rubbing bodies together. (Dry kissing is kissing with closed mouths.) People can do all of these things as much as they like without increasing their chance of spreading or catching HIV. Masturbation is also a form of safe sex.

Sexual acts with low risk of spreading HIV

Many people ask whether kissing can spread HIV. Kissing has never been shown to spread HIV. However, people with HIV can have the virus in their saliva, so there may be a small chance of spreading HIV through kissing with open mouths and touching tongues ("wet" kissing).

Oral sex is touching someone's vagina, penis, or anus with one's mouth or tongue. Oral sex can spread the virus, but HIV is spread much less often during oral sex than during anal and vaginal sex. The less semen or vaginal fluid a person's mouth touches, the less likely he will get HIV. This means using a condom on the penis or a covering (plastic wrap or latex) on the vagina will lower the chance of HIV being spread. Oral sex on a woman is probably less safe during her period or menses.

Vaginal, anal, and oral sex with a condom are not completely safe, but they are much safer than not using a condom. There is some risk even when condoms are used, because they can break or leak. To lower this risk, a man can use a condom but ejaculate outside his partner's vagina, anus, or mouth.

Sexual acts with high risk of spreading HIV

Vaginal sex frequently spreads HIV. Semen, vaginal fluid, and blood can be exchanged during vaginal or anal sex. A woman has a higher chance of getting HIV during vaginal sex than a man does. In other words, a woman having vaginal sex with a man who has HIV is more at risk than a man who has vaginal sex with a woman who has HIV. The risk is probably twice as great. It may be because more semen gets inside a woman's vagina than vaginal fluid enters a man's penis. There may also be more virus in semen than in vaginal fluid.

Anal sex spreads HIV even more easily than vaginal sex. This may be because the skin inside of a person's anus is more fragile than the skin inside of a woman's vagina. It may tear and bleed. The same risk for spreading HIV exists for anal sex between two men as for anal sex between a man and a woman. As with vaginal sex, the "receptive" partner in anal sex has double the "insertive" partner's risk of getting HIV. Who is having anal sex does not matter. It is anal sex that puts people at risk.

How to avoid spreading HIV through sex

There are five general ways to make sex safer. These are:

1. Choose carefully and limit the number of sexual partners.
2. Get tested and treated for sexually transmitted diseases, and ask partners to get tested and treated too.
3. Have safer types of sex.
4. Use condoms or other barriers during sex.
5. Have sex less frequently.

Choose carefully and limit the number of sexual partners

A person who lives in an area where many people have HIV has a higher chance of having HIV himself. There is also a high chance that the next person he has sex with will have the virus. The chances that his partner will have HIV depend on whether she has done something that puts her at risk. Some issues to think about are whether she has had sex in the past, with whom she had sex (how many partners she has had, and what their histories were), whether she used condoms, whether she has used drugs and shared needles, and whether she

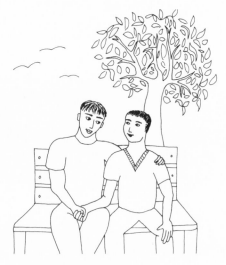

Talking to your partner could save your life and your partner's!

has had a blood transfusion. Since it is impossible to tell if people are infected by looking at them, partners need to talk about these issues before having sex. Knowing people's life stories and their risk factors for HIV can help you estimate their chances of having HIV. Talking with your partner could save your life—and hers!

People who have sex with several partners can lower their risk of getting HIV by having sex with fewer partners and having sex with people who are less likely to have HIV. Sex workers who do not always use condoms have a high risk of having HIV because they have so many partners. Someone who has had sex with a sex worker without using a condom is at risk of having HIV. There are many different names for sex workers. It does not matter what a sex worker is called, or whether the person paid for sex or was the sex worker's boyfriend, girlfriend, or spouse. The risk of HIV infection is the same. People should be encouraged not to visit sex workers or, if they do, to use condoms or take other precautions. They should ask their sex partners whether they have ever had sex with a sex worker.

Because sharing needles can spread HIV, partners should be asked whether they have ever injected drugs like heroin or speed. Asking about a partner's drug use, now and in the past, will help a person know if there is a high or low chance that the partner has HIV.

If two people choose to have sex only with each other, they are choosing to be monogamous. If neither partner already has HIV, being monogamous helps keep them both safe from HIV. They can stay safe by not having unsafe sex or sharing needles outside the relationship and not receiving transfusions of blood unless it has been tested for HIV. If they take these precautions, they can be sure of never getting HIV. They are an "HIV-sheltered" couple.

If neither partner has ever had sex, shared needles, or had a blood transfusion, then there is no chance that either person has HIV. However, if just one of these things is *not* true for either partner, there is a chance that he could have HIV, and he should be tested. Since many people have had sex by the time they choose to build a monogamous relationship, in order to be sure that a negative HIV test really means that there is no virus, a month must pass after the last chance of getting HIV (see Chapter 7, "HIV testing"). Until this has happened and they can be sure the test is

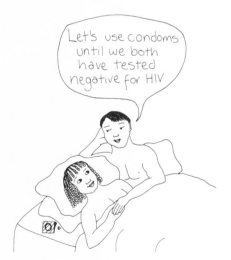

Let's use condoms until we both have tested negative for HIV

accurate, even partners in a monogamous relationship should use condoms and take other precautions. To become an HIV-sheltered couple, most people will need to be tested. After the second test, two people without HIV who only have sex with each other could have sex without condoms forever and be sure of never getting HIV from sex.

Sometimes people who think of themselves as monogamous have sex with people outside their "monogamous" relationship. When this happens, even if both partners tested negative for HIV in the past, they are no longer an HIV-sheltered couple. This is why it is very important for people to tell their partners if they have sex outside the relationship. People in a polygamous relationship (having more than one sexual partner) can also be sheltered from HIV as long as all of the partners do not have HIV and do not have unsafe sex outside the relationship or engage in other risky behavior.

Encourage people to talk with their partners about which sexual practices have no risk, low risk, or a high risk of spreading HIV. People can practice safer acts like kissing, rubbing, and oral sex rather than vaginal or anal sex. This is especially important when one of the partners has HIV or is at a high risk of having HIV.

When one person in a faithful couple is infected with HIV

Sometimes one person in a committed couple has HIV, and the partner does not. This is surprisingly common. Counseling people in a couple like this (sometimes called a discordant couple) can be difficult. One or both people in the couple may not believe the results of the tests—especially if they have been together and faithful for some time. Or the person who does not have HIV may blame the other for bringing HIV into the relationship. People may be afraid to be tested because this situation is so uncomfortable for most couples. Support from a counselor, friends, and family can help a discordant couple deal with the challenge of having HIV.

Discordant couples often question how it is possible for one of them to have HIV and the other not. Many things may be part of the answer—how much virus the HIV-infected person has, what kind of sex the couple has—but the main answer is chance. Chance means it is possible to get HIV the first time you have sex with an infected person and it is possible to have sex many times with that person and not get infected.

In a discordant couple the strategy of "being faithful" is not much help for preventing the spread of HIV. But it can be challenging to encourage people in a faithful, monogamous relationship (or in committed polygamous relationships) to use condoms or to practice abstinence or safer sex. Sometimes a couple may also believe marriage means each person is meant to share the fate of the other—even HIV—and there is no point trying to avoid it. Discordant couples can form support groups to discuss these issues. People in a support group can sometimes convince others that having sex in ways that protect the uninfected partner, like using condoms, is possible and worthwhile.

STD treatment helps stop HIV from spreading

A group of health workers and researchers in Mwanza, Tanzania studied twelve villages near Lake Victoria to find out whether treating people with STDs would help stop the spread of HIV. In six villages, health workers at local clinics received special training and drugs for the treatment of STDs. In the other six villages, normal STD programs were continued. At the end of the project, the villages with the supported STD treatment programs had 40% fewer new cases of HIV infection!

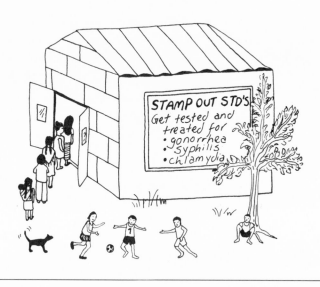

Get tested and treated for sexually transmitted diseases

HIV is spread through sex. People get other sexually transmitted diseases (STDs) like syphilis, gonorrhea, herpes, chlamydia, and chancroid the same way. This means people at risk for HIV are also at risk for these diseases. If someone has an STD, it greatly increases her risk of getting or spreading HIV. This is because these diseases cause sores and inflammation. The good news is that syphilis, gonorrhea, chlamydia, and chancroid can all be treated. To stop the spread of these diseases and to greatly lower the chance of getting HIV or giving it to someone else, people should be tested for STDs and treated.

Have safer types of sex

Some types of sex have no chance of spreading HIV; others have a high chance. Understanding the difference can help people choose safer types of sex. People can be encouraged to have oral sex instead of vaginal sex, or to touch each other with their hands instead of having oral sex. Making these choices will lower a person's risk of getting HIV.

A condom is a soft rubber shield that is placed over a man's penis. It acts like a bag that keeps semen from entering a sexual partner's body. It can be used during vaginal sex, anal sex, or oral sex. Condoms do two things at the same time—they prevent pregnancy and they prevent the spread of HIV and other STDs such as gonorrhea, syphilis, chancroid, and chlamydia.

Using condoms is important but does not guarantee absolute safety. If a condom breaks or slides off the penis, it may not prevent pregnancy, HIV, or another STD. Learning to use a condom correctly helps avoid this problem.

A condom that has been in a pocket for months may not work well because age and heat will make it break more easily. Any condom package should be opened carefully to avoid tearing the condom. Many condoms come with lubricants already inside; these can help sex with a condom feel better and they can help keep the condom from breaking. Oil-based lubricants like petroleum jelly or vegetable oil should not be used with condoms because they weaken and break them.

The "female" condom

Recently, a new type of condom was made: the "female" condom. A woman puts the female condom inside her vagina before she has sex. The advantage to a female condom is that a woman can use it without having to ask a man to put a condom on his penis. The female condom prevents the spread of HIV and other STDs, and pregnancy, just as well as the usual male condom. The problem with it is that it is expensive and not available in many places.

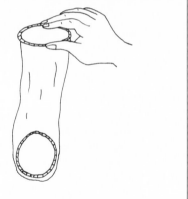

Female condom

Learning to use a condom takes practice, but once a person knows how, putting on a condom is easy. If a man has never used a condom before, he should practice putting one on alone. Rolling a condom onto your fingers, a piece of wood, or a banana is a good way to show a group of people how to use a condom. But, make sure they understand that the condom goes on the penis and not on the fingers! Helping a sexual partner put on the condom can make condom use part of sex. Some people are so skilled at putting on condoms that

How to use a condom

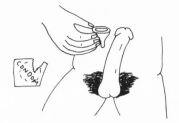

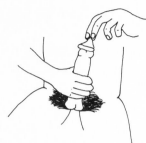

1. carefully open and remove the condom

2. use the condom when the penis is hard

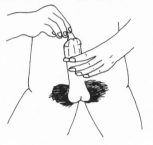

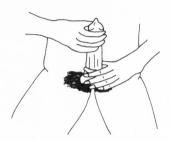

3. press air out of the tip of the condom

4. Unroll the condom to the base of the penis

their partners never notice. Some people are able to use just their mouths to put a condom on another person.

Condoms should be put on when a man's penis is hard. A condom comes rolled up in a ring and should be unrolled directly onto the penis—do not unroll it first and then try to slide it on. Always press air out of the tip and leave some space there to catch the sperm. This will help prevent the condom

Selling condoms in Kenya

In 1997, the Kenyan Department of Public Health set up condom-selling machines in the Isiolo district to help stop the spread of HIV. The condom machines were placed in public places such as bars, hotels, and lodging houses. The hope is that making condoms easier to buy will mean more people will use them.

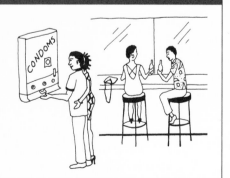

from breaking. If the condom does not fit down to the base of the penis, the man should be careful not to put the penis into his partner's body beyond the base of the condom, or it may come off inside his partner. A condom should also be taken off correctly. After a man ejaculates, he should hold on to the base of the condom before gently pulling out from his partner. This avoids spilling sperm or losing the condom inside his partner. Condoms should never be used more than once.

Condoms are usually sold in pharmacies. No doctor's prescription is needed to buy them. Often condoms can be found in other places like clinics, restaurants, bars, and hotels. Sometimes they can be bought from vending machines. Help people find the cheapest place to buy condoms. Many organizations now try to sell condoms at a low price or give them away for free in countries where they are not made; if there are health or HIV-related organizations in your area, ask if they can supply condoms.

Microbicides and spermicides

Chemicals that kill sperm are called spermicides. Sometimes condoms are coated with spermicides to increase their protection against pregnancy. Scientists are trying to develop a microbicide — a chemical that will protect against the HIV microbe — but as of 2005, they have not been successful. Several years ago, researchers thought that a microbicide called nonoxynol-9 might provide that protection, but in fact nonoxynol-9 can irritate the soft skin inside the vagina or anus so much that it should not be used.

When people ask you about condoms, bring up questions like "Who is responsible for making sure a condom is used during sex? How can you tell your partner that you want to use a condom during sex? What if your partner refuses to use a condom? Is sex without a condom so much better it is worth dying for?" Remember to talk about condoms with men *and* women.

Condoms are the most common barrier used to prevent the spread of HIV. However, people also use plastic wrap or latex sheets as a barrier during oral sex. Even though oral sex already has a low risk of spreading HIV, the risk is not zero.

Make condoms work better

Put them on and take them off properly

Do not store them in the sun, a pants pocket, or a wallet

Do not use condoms that have passed their expiration date

Use latex condoms; they prevent the spread of HIV better than ones made from lambskin

Use condoms with lubricant

Therefore, some couples, especially those where one partner is known to have HIV, use a barrier during oral sex to make sure that they do not spread the virus.

Does taking contraceptive (birth control) pills or having a contraceptive implanted under the skin (Norplant) prevent HIV infection? Studies of women in Africa showed that if women took "the pill" they were *more* likely to get HIV. This was probably because women taking the pill to prevent pregnancy were less likely to use condoms. If a woman is using the pill to prevent pregnancy, do not forget to remind her that it does not protect against HIV or other STDs. She should still practice safer sex!

Have sex less often

Whenever people have unsafe sex they risk spreading HIV. Decreasing the number of times people have sex decreases their risk of getting or giving HIV.

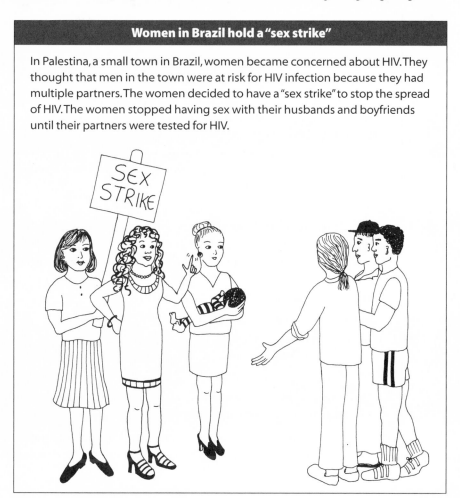

Women in Brazil hold a "sex strike"

In Palestina, a small town in Brazil, women became concerned about HIV. They thought that men in the town were at risk for HIV infection because they had multiple partners. The women decided to have a "sex strike" to stop the spread of HIV. The women stopped having sex with their husbands and boyfriends until their partners were tested for HIV.

For example, if a person has vaginal sex twenty times a month with someone with HIV, he has a higher chance of getting HIV than if he has vaginal sex four times a month.

It is hard for people to stop having sex, but it may be possible for them to lower the number of times they have sex, or to lower the number of times they have unsafe sex. If a woman's husband has many outside partners, you can suggest that she ask her husband to use condoms. She can also reduce the amount of sex that she has with her husband. This way, if he does get HIV, she will have less of a chance of becoming infected herself. If people change parts of their sexual behavior, such as how often and what type of sex they have, they can lower their risk of getting HIV. In fact, people can have sex as many times as they want without spreading HIV as long as the sexual acts are safe. Knowing this may make changing sexual behavior easier.

Will I get HIV by having sex?

Answering these questions can help people understand their risk of getting HIV.

1. What is the chance that my sexual partner has HIV?

   Does he come from a community with a lot of HIV?

   What has been his risk of getting HIV over the past ten years? (Has he had many sexual partners? Has he had unsafe sex? Has he injected drugs and shared needles? Has he had a blood transfusion?)

   What are the chances that his past sexual partners had HIV? (Did they have many sexual partners? Did they inject drugs? Were any of them sex workers?)

2. Do I or my sexual partner have a sexually transmitted disease? Syphilis, herpes, chancroid, gonorrhea, chlamydia, and other STDs increase the chance that HIV will be spread.

   Have I had pain when I urinate, or have I had pus come from the head of my penis or from my vagina?

   Do I have a sore on my vagina, penis, or anus?

   Does my partner have a sore on her vagina? On his penis?

3. What type of sex am I having with my partner? Anal and vaginal sex have a higher risk of spreading HIV than oral sex. Touching and dry kissing have no risk.

4. Do my partner and I use any barrier protection? Condoms, plastic, and latex wraps can be used to prevent the exchange of body fluids.

5. How many times have I had sex with my partner? The more frequently someone has sex with a person who has HIV, the greater the chance that HIV will be spread.

Other factors that affect the spread of HIV

People who have HIV do not seem to have the same amount of virus in their body fluids at all times. Health workers believe that people who are in the very early or very late stages of HIV infection—people who have just been infected and people who are sick with AIDS—are more likely to spread the virus than those who have HIV but no symptoms. Unfortunately, there is no easy method for finding out how much HIV is in a person's body fluids. All people with HIV, and all people whose partners may have HIV, should always take care not to spread the virus.

Answering Olga's questions

"Can I get AIDS from cleaning the rooms of German and American visitors? Should my husband and I use condoms to avoid giving each other AIDS?"

Olga is worried about AIDS but does not understand how AIDS is spread. You can help Olga by explaining that HIV is only spread by having body fluids such as blood, semen, or vaginal fluid enter the body. This means that she cannot get AIDS from cleaning the rooms of foreigners, even if they have AIDS. If neither Olga nor her husband has HIV, and if they only have sex with each other, then they do not need to use condoms during sex. They are considered an HIV-sheltered couple. You can tell Olga and her husband that they can avoid HIV in the future by not having sex with other people, by not sharing needles, and by not getting transfusions of blood that has not been tested for HIV.

6

The spread of HIV by ways other than sex

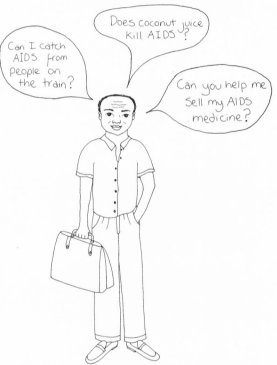

Clarence's story

Clarence is a "train doctor" in Ghana. He makes the trip from Accra to Kumasi almost every day. The people on the train rarely get to see a doctor and they ask Clarence about all kinds of health problems. He gives advice and sells soaps, vitamins, and injections to treat fevers. Many of the people riding the train have asked him if he has a cure for AIDS. He believes that one of his injections of vitamins and penicillin prevents AIDS. Clarence has heard about dirty needles spreading HIV and cleans his needles with coconut juice. He also uses a different needle for each train car. Clarence tries to buy clean needles once a month, but they are expensive and sometimes hard to get. When he hears that you are teaching people about AIDS, he asks, "Can you help me sell my AIDS medicine? Can I catch AIDS from people on the train? Does coconut juice kill AIDS?"

How HIV is spread

In most cases, people have become infected with HIV by having sex. However, there are other ways that HIV can be spread: by dirty needles and instruments, by transfusions of HIV-infected blood, and from a mother to her baby. In this chapter we discuss these other ways that HIV is spread.

HIV, alcohol, and drug use

Alcohol and drug use make it more likely that a person will get or spread HIV. This is not because HIV is in alcohol or drugs—it is not—but because people taking drugs or drinking alcohol do not think clearly and are more likely to do things that put them at risk for getting HIV. The most common way is by having unsafe sex.

Many people drink alcohol. Some people drink so much alcohol that it harms them. They are called "alcoholics." Drinking alcohol damages their bodies; it also changes the way they act, which can damage their relationships with other people and their ability to work. Other people almost never drink alcohol. When it comes to getting or spreading HIV, what matters is that

---

CAGE questions

Some people do not know that they have a problem with alcohol. If you ask someone whether she is an alcoholic, you may not hear the truth. Here are some other questions you can ask instead. These are known as the CAGE questions. If someone answers "yes" to two or more of these questions, she probably has a problem with alcohol.

C   Have you ever tried to Cut down (lower) the amount of alcohol that you drink?

A   Do you get Annoyed when people talk to you about your drinking?

G   Have you ever felt Guilty about your drinking?

E   Have you ever needed an "Eye-opener" (a drink) when you woke up in the morning to steady your nerves or prevent a headache?

---

drinking alcohol causes people to make bad decisions. For example, going to a bar to drink may lead a man to spend his money on alcohol when his children are hungry at home. After having a few drinks, he may decide to visit a sex worker—even if he knows she might have HIV.

Just like people who drink alcohol, people who use drugs are also at risk of getting HIV. People who use drugs may trade sex for drugs or money. They may want drugs so badly they have unsafe sex. Drug use is also dangerous because HIV can be spread by needles that have been used by someone else to inject drugs. A person using a dirty needle puts a little of someone else's blood into herself. If HIV is in the blood, she could get infected.

In some countries, it is against the law for people to have needles or syringes unless a doctor has prescribed them. People who use drugs like

---

Millions of people use drugs worldwide

Between 5 and 10% of the people in the world have alcohol-related disease. Two million people die each year from alcohol use. About 144 million people, almost 2.5% of the world's population, smoke marijuana or hashish. About 14 million people use cocaine, 9 million use heroin, and 29 million take amphetamine-like drugs ("speed").

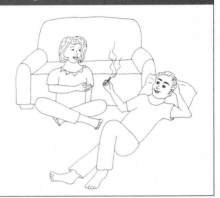

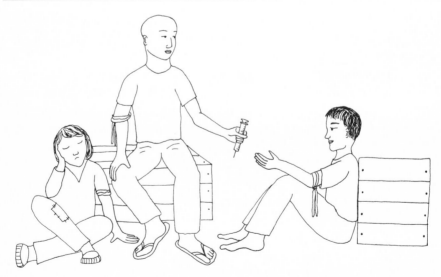

Sharing needles spreads HIV.

The spread of HIV by ways other than sex

Drug injection and HIV

Intravenous (IV) needles are used to draw blood and to give fluids and medicines. Injectionists, traditional healers, doctors, and nurses all use intravenous needles.

These needles can also be used to inject illegal drugs. People who give themselves drugs in this way are called drug injectors, injection drug users (IDU), or intravenous drug users (IVDU). HIV is spread by drug use all over the world. In some places 50% or more of all people who inject drugs have HIV.

Drug injectors can give HIV not only to other drug users, but also to their sexual partners. If a woman becomes pregnant she may give HIV to her baby. The spread of HIV among people who share needles is a problem for the drug injector, her or his sexual partner, and their children.

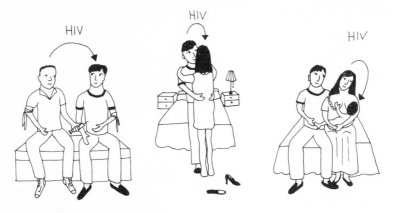

A person who has shared needles can spread HIV to his partner and their baby.

heroin or amphetamines often buy needles illegally or rent them from someone else. In New York City in the United States, people inject drugs in "shooting galleries," where people rent used needles. These needles have been used by many different people. The more people share needles, the more likely it is they will become infected with HIV.

How can drug injectors avoid HIV?

Injecting drugs does not directly cause AIDS; sharing needles with other people is what causes the spread of HIV from person to person. This is why people should avoid sharing needles, cookers (equipment used to prepare drugs for injection), cotton, or anything used to inject drugs. Drug injectors can lower their risk of getting HIV in three ways:

1. *Stop injecting drugs.* It is often hard to stop using drugs because they are addictive. People who are addicted will become sick if they do not have drugs. Although it is very difficult for drug injectors to quit using drugs, it is not impossible. You can help them. Find out if programs are available in your community for people who want to stop using drugs. Learn how people can join these programs. Get to know the people who work in the programs. There may be clinics that give methadone to drug injectors. Methadone is a drug like morphine and heroin, but it is taken by mouth and therefore does not spread HIV. Methadone gives people less of a "high" than heroin, but it lasts for 24 hours. This means people do not need a new "fix" every few hours. Since methadone is legal, they do not need to steal or have sex in order to pay for drugs.

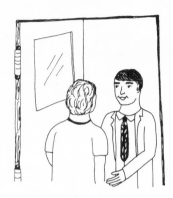

DRUG TREATMENT CENTER

2. *Use new needles.* If a drug user is unable to quit using drugs, he can avoid HIV by using only clean, new ones. Teach drug users that dirty needles spread HIV. If your community has a needle-exchange program, tell drug users that they can get clean needles for free by bringing in old ones. You might think that such a program would increase the number of people who use drugs. But in communities that have needle-exchange programs, the number of people who inject drugs has not increased—and the number of drug injectors who get HIV has decreased. (Also, people who use new, clean needles get fewer skin infections.)

3. *Use clean needles.* Sometimes getting new needles is difficult or expensive. In these situations, people can learn how to clean their needles. Everyone who shares needles should clean them between users. The most common way to clean needles is with bleach (Cloro, Clorox, etc.). Bleach kills HIV, but do not drink it or inject it, because it can hurt or kill people when inside the body. Because of this, after cleaning the needles with bleach, use clean water to wash away the bleach. People can also clean needles by boiling them in water for 30 minutes. (Also see the box on "How to clean needles and other instruments" later in this chapter.)

Cleaning Needles

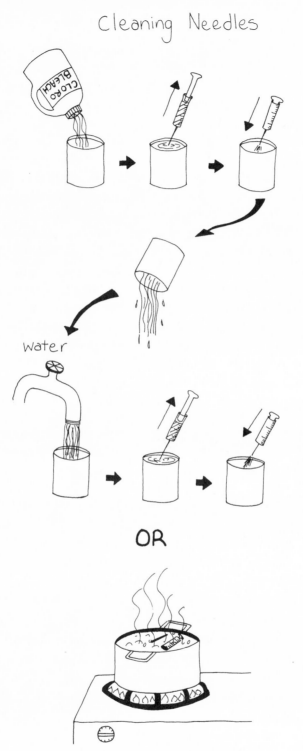

OR

Boil in water for thirty minutes

HIV and blood transfusions

Blood or blood products (such as serum or plasma) can save a person's life. However, they can also be dangerous. If blood and blood products have not been carefully "screened," or tested, a person could get several diseases, including AIDS, from them. The chances of getting HIV from blood that has not been tested depend on how many blood donors—people who give blood—have HIV. For example, in a city where 25% of the donors have HIV and screening is not available, HIV is in one of every four units of blood. HIV has been found in all parts of blood. This means that packed red blood cells, serum, plasma, and clotting factors can all contain HIV. Even in places where blood is screened carefully, there is still a very small chance that it contains HIV, viruses that cause hepatitis or malaria, or other organisms.

Many countries in the world are taking special care to keep their blood supply free of HIV. They do this first by screening donors and second by testing blood. Blood banks collect and store blood for later use. To reduce the chance that the blood contains HIV or other organisms, blood banks screen donors by asking people about their sexual and drug-use practices. People with a high risk of having HIV are then asked not to give blood. This lowers the chance that the blood supply will have HIV. Unfortunately, in areas where many people have HIV it is difficult to find donors.

Sample blood bank questionnaire

These are some questions that blood banks, clinics, and hospitals can use to screen their donors and find out who has a high risk of having HIV. A "yes" answer to even one of the questions means that the blood should not be used.

Do you have AIDS or have you had a positive test for HIV (the AIDS virus)?

Have you had sex with someone who has AIDS or who has had a positive HIV test?

Have you ever received money or drugs in exchange for sex?

Have you had sex with a sex worker?

Have you ever injected illegal drugs like heroin or speed?

Have you had sex with someone who has injected illegal drugs?

Have you ever received a blood transfusion?

Are you a man who has had sex with another man?

Do you feel ill today?

People who are paid to give blood are more likely to have HIV than people who give blood for free. This is because people who want money for donating blood may not tell the truth about their risk of having HIV. They may also be more likely to have used drugs, to have exchanged sex for money, or to have had sex with someone who had HIV. People should never be paid for donating blood.

In addition to questioning donors, blood banks should test donated blood for HIV. Blood that has HIV should be thrown away. The HIV test is very accurate except during the few weeks between when people get the virus and when their bodies begin to produce antibodies. During this time, a person can test negative even though she has the virus. (For more about HIV testing, see Chapters 7 and 8.) In areas where donors are screened and blood is tested, the number of people who get HIV from blood transfusions has gone down.

The risks and benefits of giving a patient a blood transfusion should be carefully weighed. "Topping off," or giving a person extra blood to make him feel better, is a bad idea. No matter how well the blood is screened, there is still a very small chance of getting HIV. Before giving a transfusion, doctors should think very carefully about whether the person truly needs blood. Most hospitals now give blood to people less often than they did ten years ago. Sometimes a transfusion is needed to save a person's life, and in that case the benefits of receiving blood outweigh the risks of getting HIV. Learn how blood is screened in your area and ask what the chance is that a unit of blood has HIV.

Of course, there is no risk of getting HIV from *giving* blood as long as clean needles are used. You can encourage people who do not have HIV to donate blood. This adds to the blood supply and prevents the spread of HIV.

The blood supply in India

In India, most blood banks were not testing blood for HIV or other viruses. Then it was found that many blood donors had HIV. In 1996, the Indian government wrote new laws to try to make the blood supply safer. The new laws said that blood banks had to have licenses and had to test donated blood. The new laws also said that blood banks could not pay donors for their blood, so that people at high risk for infections would not give blood to get money.

There are ways to reduce the risks of getting HIV from a transfusion. One way is to have a person give her own blood a few weeks before an operation. Then her blood will be available if a transfusion is needed. This is the safest way to get a transfusion. But often there is not enough time or space in the blood bank for a pre-donation.

How to reduce the risk of spreading HIV through blood transfusions

Choosing donors

Teach health care workers about the risk of spreading HIV through blood transfusions.

Use a questionnaire to screen out high-risk donors.

Use blood from donors who give it for free, not from donors who are paid.

Use a person's own blood when possible.

Use donors with a low risk of having HIV.

Screening donated blood

Test all blood donations for HIV.

If all blood cannot be tested, other screening options can be used. For example, samples from ten donations can be pooled (combined) and tested. If the test is positive, the ten donations can then be individually tested, or all ten can be thrown away. A negative test means that all ten are safe.

Medical practices

Do not give transfusions unless absolutely necessary.

When possible, use blood expanders such as saline instead of blood.

Heat-treat blood products like plasma and clotting factors in order to kill HIV.

People often believe that getting blood from a family member is safer than getting blood from an unknown (anonymous) donor. However, this is usually *not* true, because family members may be more likely to cover up that they are at a high risk of having HIV. For example, a woman may be embarrassed to tell her family that she had sex with someone outside of her marriage.

HIV in the clinic

HIV can be spread in the clinic by needles and instruments (scalpels, forceps, scissors, specula, etc.) that have been used to give people medicine, draw blood, perform an examination, or perform surgery. Especially in an area where many people have HIV, the virus can

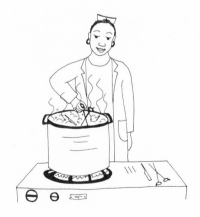

How to clean needles and other instruments

Heat methods	Time needed
Boiling	30 minutes
Steam	30 minutes
Dry-heat oven, 77°C or 170°F	30 minutes

The following chemicals can be used to clean needles and other instruments. The instruments should be rinsed with water and then soaked for at least 30 minutes in one of these solutions. Instruments should be placed in a clean area and allowed to dry before use.

Chemicals that inactivate HIV	Concentration
Sodium hypochloride (bleach)	0.5%
Sodium hydroxide	30 mM
Glutaraldehyde	2%
Formalin	4%
Paraformaldehyde	1%
Hydrogen peroxide	6%
Ethyl peroxide	1%
Lysol (household cleaner)	1%
NP-40 detergent	1%
Chlorhexidine gluconate/ethanol	4/25%
Ammonia	1:1 (ammonia to water)
Isopropyl alcohol	50%
Chloramine	2%
Ethanol	70%
Polyvidone iodine	2.5%

None of these works inside a person's body!

spread quickly if needles and instruments are used on more than one patient. However, most health workers know that HIV can be spread in this way, so they either do not use needles a second time or they clean all needles and instruments before using them on another patient. If simple measures are taken, spread of HIV in hospitals and clinics should be rare.

Avoiding HIV in the clinic

When people ask your advice about how to avoid getting HIV when they visit the doctor or other health care worker, you can tell them to:

Ask for new or sterilized instruments.

Go to health care workers who clean needles using the methods described in this chapter (not, for example, with coconut juice).

Ask the doctor or health care worker if it is possible to take pills instead of injections.

Use sterilized instruments if you are piercing your ears or getting a tattoo.

Ask health care workers to use new, clean gloves when doing procedures that may spill body fluids.

How can health workers avoid getting or spreading HIV on the job?

People who take care of people with HIV often worry about getting the virus from patients. Procedures such as giving injections, drawing blood, doing pelvic examinations (examining a woman's vagina and cervix), and performing surgery usually involve some contact with body fluids. However, if normal safety measures are followed, there should be very little risk of getting HIV for the health care worker or the patient. (The box called "Are you at risk" gives some questions that can help health care workers find out their risk of getting or spreading HIV in the clinic.)

Are you at risk for getting HIV at work?

How much contact do you have with body fluids?

What are you doing now to prevent contact with body fluids?

Do you protect yourself all the time or only sometimes?

How do you clean instruments? Do you sterilize them?

Do you reuse syringes or do you throw them away?

Do you have a safe place to put sharp, dirty instruments?

Are clean gloves available?

If the workplace is unsafe, how can you make it safer?

A pelvic examination with a dirty instrument can give a woman HIV. Clean instruments and gloves should be used by people at all times when in contact with body fluid (during pelvic examinations, when using a needle to draw blood, and during surgery). It is best if gloves are used once and then thrown out. Some rubber gloves are made to be reused; these gloves should be steril-

It is very rare to get HIV after being stuck by a needle—about 1 in 300 people who are stuck by a needle that has been used on a person with HIV will become infected. There are some things that increase the chance that a person will get HIV from a needle injury:

if the injury is deep and in a muscle

if there was patient's blood in the needle

if the patient has AIDS (this may mean there is more virus in the patient's blood than if she just had HIV)

ized after each use in one of the solutions listed in the box "How to kill HIV." If no gloves are available, then health workers should carefully wash their hands immediately after contact with each patient. They should also keep their fingernails short and cover any open sores on their hands with waterproof plaster, tape, or bandages. Tables and floors should be washed with a bleach solution every day *and* after each examination or procedure. People doing this job should wear gloves, because they may touch body fluids. If you only have dirty instruments, think about whether the risk of spreading HIV is greater than the benefit of the examination or procedure. It may be better not to treat the patient.

Needles that are thrown away with paper waste or linens can cause injuries. Needles and other sharp instruments should be thrown away in a special box called a "sharps box" or "sharps container." The box should be made of a material that is thick and strong enough that the needles and other instruments cannot pierce it. You can buy sharps containers that are made of plastic, or you can use a strong cardboard box with a small

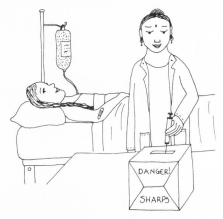

hole in the top. Label all sharps containers so people do not open them by mistake and hurt themselves. Whoever uses a needle should drop it in the sharps container immediately after using it. Needles should not be left lying around—needles and other sharp instruments that are hidden on trays cluttered with cotton swabs and papers can be deadly. And do not put the cap back on a needle; many injuries have happened this way.

How to prevent injuries when using needles, scalpels, and other sharp instruments

In the clinic

Do not

    put caps back on needles

    bend or break needles

Do

    remove used needles from your work area

    put needles and other sharp instruments in "sharps boxes" after using them

    keep sharps boxes near where work is being done

    wear gloves when using a needle to draw blood (if you stick yourself after drawing blood from a patient, the glove will clean some of the patient's blood off the needle before the needle punctures your skin)

    use protective barriers such as gloves, gowns, masks, and eyewear (glasses or safety glasses) when a lot of contact with body fluids is expected

    wash hands immediately if they have body fluid on them, and also wash them after seeing each patient

In surgery

Pass sharp instruments back into a tray and not into an open hand

Always say "needle back" or "sharps back" when passing these instruments back

Bandage all cuts and nicks on hands before putting on gloves

Wear a double pair of gloves

If blood or other body fluid gets under a glove, take off gloves immediately, scrub hands, and put on new, clean gloves

Think safety!

If someone is cut with a dirty instrument or needle, she should clean the wound immediately with soap and water. If a person is stuck by a needle that has HIV-infected blood on it, her chance of becoming infected with HIV is about 1 in 300. This is high enough to mean that everyone should take precautions very seriously, but low enough that spread of HIV in the health care setting remains rare.

HIV outside the clinic

People use needles for injecting medicines outside of the clinic or hospital. For example, people with diabetes inject medicine at home. In Ivory Coast,

All over the world people get tattoos and scars. If the needles, razor blades, or knives used to make the marks are not clean, HIV can be spread from one person to another. In some parts of the world people pierce parts of their bodies and put in pieces of jewelry. HIV can spread if the piercing instruments used are not cleaned properly. HIV can also be spread through the use of acupuncture needles if they are not sterilized before reuse.

In some parts of the world, people circumcise boys and girls before they reach adulthood. Circumcision for a boy means that the foreskin is cut off of the tip of the penis. "Circumcision" or "genital mutilation" for a girl means that the clitoris and/or vaginal lips are cut off. Sometimes the vagina is sewn up. Circumcisions are performed either in the hospital or clinic, or in the community. If instruments are not cleaned, HIV can be spread.

people travel from village to village selling injections and medicines. In Mexico, some people have small stores where they inject vitamins and antibiotics and other medicines. These people are known as "injectionists." You can talk with injectionists and see what they know about HIV and the problems with using dirty needles. Talk with them about ways to clean needles.

Mothers, babies, and HIV

HIV can pass from a mother to her baby during pregnancy, birth, or breast-feeding. Without antiretroviral medicines or other prevention, about one of every three babies born to women with HIV is infected with the virus during the pregnancy or birth. The chance of a mother passing the virus on to her baby can be reduced greatly if she takes antiretroviral medicines throughout the last 3 months of her pregnancy or during birth. See the section "Medicines for HIV" in the appendix to learn how to give these medicines.

The best way to prevent the spread of HIV to children is to protect mothers from getting HIV in the first place. See Chapter 5 and Chapter 12 for how to help women and their partners prevent the spread of HIV.

If a woman already has HIV and does not want to become pregnant or risk giving birth to a child with HIV, she can use contraceptives (birth control) to prevent pregnancy. Some common contraceptives are condoms, contraceptive pills, injections (Depo-Provera), diaphragms, intrauterine devices (IUDs), and implants. Condoms are the only of these methods that can prevent the spread of HIV too. Some couples have sex only around the time of the woman's period because she is much less likely to get pregnant at that time. This does not work well unless the couple keeps very careful track of which days the woman can become pregnant. Couples can also avoid pregnancy by having oral sex or by touching each other in sexual ways instead of having sexual intercourse.

If a woman with HIV does become pregnant, she may think about having an abortion. Performed correctly, abortions are safe procedures. However, in some communities abortion is illegal and some communities do not have the means to do safe abortions. Having children may be so important to the woman or her family that she may choose to have children even though there is a risk of passing HIV. This is a complicated decision and many people including the woman's family and community will have opinions about what she should do.

When a woman with HIV gives birth, it is difficult to know whether the baby has HIV. All babies born to mothers with HIV have HIV antibodies in their blood because these antibodies are transmitted from the mother to the baby during pregnancy. HIV tests check for HIV antibodies, so all babies of HIV positive mothers test positive. This does not mean that all the babies have HIV. After 15–18 months, the mother's antibodies will all have left the baby's body and the baby's HIV test will be accurate. Many babies that have HIV will become sick in the first year or two of life. Some, however, grow to be children, living many years with HIV.

Breastfeeding and HIV

Breast milk is the best food for young babies. It is more nutritious, safer, and cheaper than bottled milk or baby formula. Breast milk also protects the baby against disease. Babies who are breastfed have a better chance of staying healthy and living longer.

Unfortunately, mothers with HIV can pass the infection to their babies through breast milk. No one knows why HIV is passed to some babies and not others, but HIV probably passes more easily during breastfeeding when:

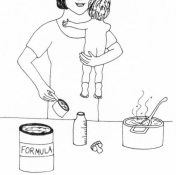

- the mother recently became infected with HIV.
- the mother is very sick with AIDS.
- the mother gives formula, teas, or other fluids along with breast milk.
- the mother has cracked nipples or a breast infection.
- the baby has thrush in her mouth.

For most mothers, even mothers with HIV, breastfeeding is the safest way to feed their babies. That is because in most places formula and other milks cause many babies to get sick or die from diarrhea or hunger. Many more babies die from taking formula than get sick or die from HIV passed through breastfeeding. If a mother with HIV chooses to breastfeed, here are some things that may make it safer:

- Give only breast milk for the first 6 months. Babies who have breast milk and formula, teas, or other foods or drinks are more likely to become infected than babies who drink only breast milk. Any other foods or liquids will irritate the baby's intestines.
- Stop breastfeeding completely after 6 months.
- Position the baby correctly to avoid cracked nipples.
- Treat thrush, cracked nipples, and breast infections right away.
- Do not feed the baby from a breast that has mastitis or an abscess—instead, remove the milk and throw it away.

A woman who is being treated with medicines for HIV is less likely to pass the disease while breastfeeding.

A baby that is fed only formula has no chance of getting HIV from breast milk. So if formula can be given safely, it is the best option. But it is only safe when the family has enough money to afford enough formula, clean water to mix the formula with, and fuel to boil and sterilize bottles.

Families who give formula must follow the directions on the package — exactly. Do not thin the formula by adding extra water or by using less milk or powder. Dirty bottles and nipples or watered-down formula can kill a baby.

Misunderstandings about HIV

Many people worry about getting HIV. For example, in one town in the United States, parents banded together to stop a nine-year-old child with HIV from going to school because they thought their children could get HIV in school. We know there is no risk to children who go to school with another child who has HIV; but whenever a new disease is found, fear and a lack of information will cause some people to have false ideas about the disease.

People who are ill should be cared for with kindness. This is true whether someone has cancer, diabetes, or AIDS. In the past, people with cancer were sometimes treated unfairly. Even though cancer is not spread from person to person, some people lost their jobs and their friends when it was known that they had cancer. People with cancer had these difficulties for social reasons, not biological ones. This is also the case with HIV. Even though it is an infectious disease, HIV can spread from person to person in only a few ways. We must all take care not to let fear of HIV and AIDS make us treat people unfairly.

Answering Clarence's questions

"Can you help me sell my AIDS medicine? Can I catch AIDS from people on the train? Does coconut juice kill AIDS?"

Clarence has some important questions about AIDS. He knows a little about AIDS , but he also has some false information. Because he treats so many people on the train, it is important for him to understand how HIV is spread. He needs to understand that HIV can be spread from person to person through dirty needles. Clarence thinks that he can stop people from getting AIDS with an injection of penicillin and vitamins. This is a dangerous idea. If people believe Clarence, they will think they can have unsafe sex or share needles with someone with HIV and still not get the virus. There is no injection that will stop someone from getting HIV. You might try talking about this with Clarence. Over time, he could help you teach people on the train about HIV.

Cleaning needles with coconut juice does not get rid of HIV. It is best to use a new needle for each injection. However, using bleach to carefully clean needles and syringes will also work. If there is no bleach, needles and syringes should be cleaned with alcohol after each *person*, not each train car.

The only way Clarence could get HIV from someone on the train is if he sticks himself with a dirty needle. You can explain to him that using gloves, not putting caps back on needles, and putting dirty needles in a sharps container will help protect him from HIV.

HIV testing

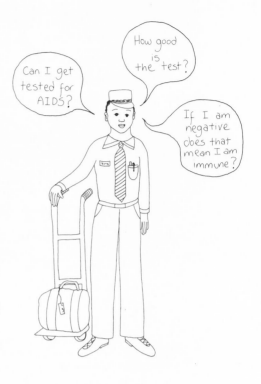

Jean-Patrice's story

Jean-Patrice is nineteen years old and lives in Cayenne, the capital of French Guiana. He moved to Cayenne six months ago from his village in the southern rainforest, where he was a farmer. Now he works in a hotel near the center of Cayenne. He enjoys living in the city and has had several girlfriends, but he wants to earn enough money to go back to his village and start a family. Jean-Patrice has not visited his village since he moved to Cayenne. Next weekend he will return there to bring medicines to his sick mother. He is looking forward to spending time with Michelle, his girlfriend in the village, but he is worried: his doctor warned him that he may have gotten something from his last girlfriend. A friend of his has AIDS and is now very sick. Jean-Patrice comes to your clinic and asks, "Can I get tested for AIDS? How good is the test? If I am negative, does that mean I am immune?"

The HIV test

The HIV test will tell if the HIV virus is in a person's body. It does not tell that a person has AIDS. It is important to know if a person is infected with HIV so:

1. People who know they are infected can begin to take more care with nutrition, clean water, and other ways of staying healthy right away. They may also start taking certain medicines. These steps will keep people with HIV healthier for longer.
2. People who know they are infected can access care and support services available to people with HIV.
3. People who are infected can protect others and avoid passing the virus.
4. People who are infected can protect themselves so they do not get re-infected in the future.

People who wait until they are sick to get tested will have more difficulty treating their sicknesses and living healthy and positive lives.

Types of HIV tests

When a virus, bacteria, or parasite enters a person's body, the immune system begins to make antibodies that try to fight off the virus or other invader. The most common HIV tests—the rapid test, the ELISA (enzyme-linked immunosorbent assay) and the Western Blot—work by looking for antibodies to HIV.

The tests are used millions of times each year. Each has its benefits and drawbacks; because of this, the tests may be used together.

Not all tests look for antibodies. Some tests look for the virus itself. For example, one type of test involves trying to grow HIV in the laboratory from a sample of a person's blood. If the virus grows from the blood, it means the person has HIV. This type of test is difficult and expensive, and it does not always find the virus in people who are infected. Other tests, such as the nucleic acid test and the polymerase chain reaction (PCR), which look for HIV RNA or DNA, are also expensive and are rarely used.

The **CD4 T-cell count** is not an HIV test. It does not check for HIV. This test counts the number of CD4 T-cells in one microliter of blood. The CD4 cells are white blood cells that are part of the immune system. These cells help the body find and fight bacteria and viruses. When the immune system has many CD4 cells it is more able to fight off infection. CD4 cells are also

Vaccines use antibodies to prevent illness. They help a person make antibodies to fight diseases that she may come into contact with later. For example, the injected polio vaccine is made of pieces of the polio virus. These pieces are not harmful to people because they are not the whole virus. When given this vaccine, a person's body makes antibodies to the virus. If the person is infected later with the real polio virus, the antibodies will attach themselves to the virus and make it easier for the body to get rid of it. Unfortunately, there is no vaccine for HIV.

attacked and destroyed by HIV. When the number of CD4 cells in the body decreases, the immune system is less able to fight infections. The CD4 count measures how strong the immune system is.

How HIV tests work

For a rapid test, a little blood is mixed with a chemical solution. A test stick is dipped into the mixture. If the blood contains HIV antibodies, a mark on the stick will indicate that the person has HIV. This test is simple and inexpensive. They are quite accurate and the results are usually available within an hour.

There are several different types of ELISA tests. We will discuss an ELISA test that uses beads. Laboratories in your country may use a slightly different test. However, all ELISA tests are based on the same idea; they look for antibodies, and if you understand how one works you can understand the others.

A small sample of blood is separated into serum (yellow liquid) and red blood cells. Antibodies are found in the serum.

Serum is placed in a container with a round bead that has bits of HIV attached to it. If there are antibodies to HIV in the serum, they will recognize

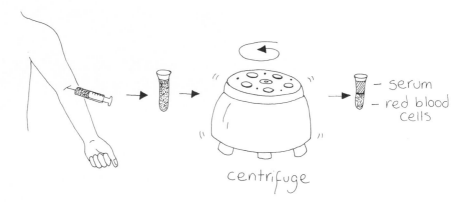

centrifuge

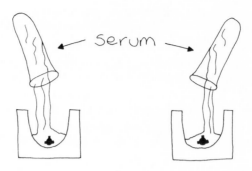

serum

serum is placed in the container
with a round bead that has pieces
of the virus attached to it

The beads are washed
If there are antibodies to HIV in
the serum they will recognize the
HIV and attach themselves to the bead

Goat antibodies are added;
they will only stick if antibodies
to HIV are present

A chemical is added and
color appears if goat and HIV
antibodies are present

 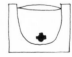

the test   the test
is   is
positive   negative

the HIV and attach themselves to the bead. Then the bead is washed. After washing, only antibodies to HIV will stick to the bead; antibodies to other viruses will be washed away.

Special antibodies taken from goat blood are then added. These antibodies attach themselves to any human antibodies that are on the virus-coated bead. The bead is washed again, and a chemical is added that brings out color in any goat antibodies that are still attached to the bead. If color appears, it means there were HIV antibodies in the person's serum. This is a positive test. If a person does not have HIV, there would be no human antibodies for the goat antibodies to attach themselves to. The goat antibodies would have been washed away and there would be no color. This is a negative test.

ELISA tests are excellent at finding antibodies against HIV. This ability to detect antibodies is called "sensitivity"; it is a basic quality of any medical test. The ELISA test for HIV is not too expensive compared to other medical tests (each test costs US$5–10). Clinics and blood banks usually use the ELISA test as a first round for testing blood.

Fingerstick and oral swab tests

The most common way to test for HIV is to examine a person's blood. People do not like to give blood, however, and collecting it can be expensive. Because of this there are now accurate tests that use a finger stick to get a little blood. Also, there is an HIV test has been made that uses a small sample from the inside of the mouth. This test is painless and is safer than a blood test because no needles are used. Unfortunately, the test is expensive and may not be available in your area.

The problem with rapid and ELISA tests is that they can make mistakes. Because they are so sensitive, they can give a positive result for blood that does not actually have HIV. This is known as a "false positive." To avoid this, most clinics and blood banks run a second test on blood that is positive on rapid and ELISA tests. They use another ELISA test or a test like the Western blot. The Western blot also looks for antibodies to HIV; it is not as sensitive, but it is able to look more closely at *what kind of* antibodies are present. It will almost never show a blood sample to be positive if it does not contain antibodies to HIV. Thus, when a Western blot is positive, a person almost always has HIV. This ability to be right when a test is positive is called "specificity," because the test is finding antibodies to a specific disease. The problem with the Western blot is that it is expensive (each test costs US$25–50). In summary, the rapid and ELISA tests have excellent sensitivity but not very good specificity, whereas the Western blot has excellent specificity but not very good sensitivity.

When to test and when not to test

When people come to you for testing, it is important to talk to them first about their individual situations. In some areas of the world, HIV infection is so common there are very few false positives. In these areas, the test is useful for most people who want to be tested. In other areas, HIV infection is rare, and it is important to ask a few questions about risk factors before testing people. If a person is at very low risk for having HIV, it might be better not to test her. There are several reasons for this. First, it may be better to use money and other resources to test people who are at high risk, not low risk. Second, if a person is at very low risk, a positive test is likely to be a false positive. To find out for sure if he has HIV, you will need to test the person a second time, with a more expensive test. Finally, getting a positive test result can make a person frightened and upset; if the result is a false positive, the person will have been frightened and upset for no reason.

What does a test result mean?

Because the body takes a couple of weeks to produce antibodies to HIV, an HIV test may be negative for up to 3 weeks after a person becomes infected. So a negative result from an ELISA test means that a person does not have HIV—*if*, in the several weeks before testing, he did not do anything that would put him at risk (for example, he did not have unsafe sex or share needles). A negative test does *not* mean that a person cannot get HIV in the future. A positive result from *both* a rapid or ELISA *and* Western blot means that a person most likely has HIV.

Sometimes the Western blot gives an answer that is not positive or negative but "indeterminate" (unclear or uncertain). Someone with an indeterminate Western blot is more likely to have HIV than someone with a negative Western blot, but less likely to have HIV than someone with a positive Western blot. Sometimes a Western blot is indeterminate because a person has only just begun to produce antibodies to HIV. But the Western blot can also be indeterminate for people who are not infected with HIV, especially if they have certain other diseases. The sensitivity and specificity of a Western blot also depend on the skills of the people performing the test. People with indeterminate tests should take another test in one month to determine if they have HIV.

A fisherman in a boat on a small lake is trying to catch tilapia. He can use either a net or a fishing pole. What he catches will depend on which tool he uses.

The net would catch all the tilapia, but it would also catch many other fish that the fisherman does not want. The net has high sensitivity because it catches all the tilapia. The net, however, has low specificity because the fisherman catches many fish in the net that are not tilapia.

The same fisherman may choose to use a fishing pole to catch tilapia. With a pole he can use bait that is only eaten by tilapia. The pole has high specificity because it only catches the kind of fish the fisherman wants. Unfortunately, the fishing pole has low sensitivity; it cannot catch all the tilapia in the lake.

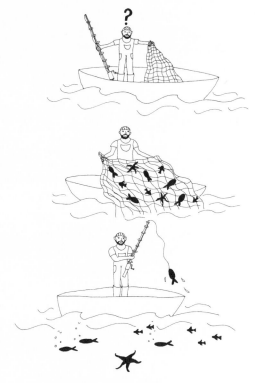

The HIV test is trying to "catch" antibodies to identify if a person has the HIV virus.

Like the net, rapid serological tests and the ELISA test for HIV have high sensitivity. They identify almost everyone who has antibodies to HIV. But these tests have low specificity which means sometimes results are positive for people who do not have HIV antibodies. If a person has a positive rapid or ELISA test but does not truly have HIV, the test is called a false positive.

Like the fishing pole, the Western blot test has high specificity because almost everyone it identifies really has antibodies to HIV. With good specificity, there are few false positives. Tests with good specificity usually have low sensitivity. They do not catch everyone who has HIV. If a person has a negative test but really does have HIV, the test is called a false negative.

It is best to have a test with both high sensitivity and high specificity, but this is not always possible. This trade-off between sensitivity and specificity in a medical test is common. Rapid serological tests and ELISA tests have good sensitivity and are used as a first test to identify all the people who have HIV antibodies-along with a few who do not. Blood samples with positive ELISA results can then be tested with a Western blot, which has good specificity. The Western blot screens out the false positives — those that are not truly infected with HIV.

The HIV test and babies

The ELISA and Western blot tests do not work for babies younger than fifteen months. This is because antibodies against HIV pass from the mother to the baby and stay in the baby's blood for about fifteen months. This means a baby can have antibodies to HIV even if she does not have the virus. If a baby being tested is at least fifteen months old, then a positive HIV test is likely to be a true positive. By the time the baby is this age, any antibodies in her blood are her own, not her mother's. For babies less than 15 months old a negative HIV test is accurate. To be sure that a positive test is correct, a test called a polymerase chain reaction (PCR) must be used.

Confidential and anonymous testing

Most people want the results of their HIV tests to be private. Telling supportive people that you have HIV can be very helpful. The right people can offer support, love, or vital services. But if a person's HIV results are shared without her consent or knowledge, this information can be used to harm her. A woman may be beaten or kicked out of her home. She may be fired from her job or shunned by her community.

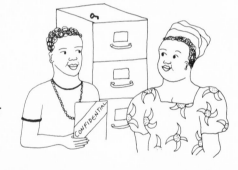

To protect a person's privacy, HIV tests should be anonymous or confidential. The test is the same for a confidential or anonymous test. The only difference is in the records kept about the results.

Confidential testing is done by a health worker who knows the name of the person being tested and the test results. The health worker keeps both private, so that other people do not know the results. Records are kept of the results and may be shared with other health workers who are involved with the person's health care.

Anonymous testing is when a health worker does not know the name of the person being tested. A number or a fake name is given to the person being tested, and the same number or name is attached to the blood sample. The person then gives their number or fake name to get the results.

Confidential testing helps limit the number of people who know about a test result. One good thing about confidential testing is that because the

HIV, blood, and pregnancy

Before a baby is born, the baby shares the mother's blood. Before the mother's blood passes to the baby, it is filtered (cleaned) by the placenta. The placenta is sometimes able to filter out HIV. This is why some babies born to mothers with HIV do not have the virus. However, the placenta is not able to filter out antibodies. This means that if a pregnant woman has HIV, she will pass her HIV antibodies to her baby. This will not hurt the baby, but it will make it difficult to test the baby for HIV infection. Over time, the antibodies in the baby fade away. If a baby still has HIV antibodies after fifteen months of age, then he is probably truly infected.

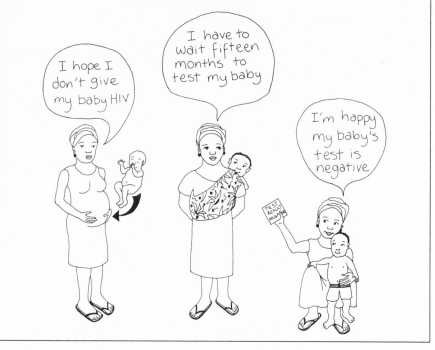

name of the person is known, a health worker can contact a person who is positive and offer further advice and treatment, even if the person does not come for a return appointment.

One problem with confidential testing is that it does not always keep information from being shared. This is why anonymous testing is sometimes used instead. If no one knows the person being tested, then it is impossible for anyone except that person to find out the results.

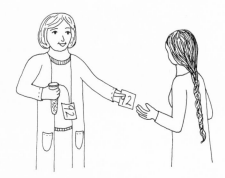

Mandatory testing

In some countries all people, or certain groups of people, are forced to be tested for HIV. This is called mandatory testing. Groups of people sometimes tested without their consent include factory workers, workers in the tourism industry, soldiers, sex workers, prisoners, immigrants, and pregnant women.

Mandatory HIV testing violates a person's right to privacy and the right to make her own decisions about her medical care. Mandatory testing often means the government or an employer unfairly controls what happens to the person after the testing. People may lose their jobs or their family support or suffer from other discrimination. People afraid of mandatory testing may avoid seeking needed health care.

There are ways to make testing both voluntary and more routine, such as offering testing in more places — hospitals, primary care clinics and people's homes, for example.

Mandatory screening

Many countries use HIV tests to screen donated blood, blood products, and organs for transplants. This is one kind of mandatory testing that is important, because it helps make sure that blood transfusions and transplants will not spread HIV.

Behavior change

There are many reasons why people think they might have HIV. These can range from knowing for sure that they are at risk because a sexual partner has AIDS to thinking they got the virus from a public toilet. When people are concerned enough to ask to be tested for HIV, they are usually eager to learn more about the virus.

The decision to be tested for HIV is often difficult (for more about counseling people who are being tested, see Chapter 8). People may be afraid of the test result, worried about who might find out the result, and concerned about how the result might change their life. The time spent waiting for test results can cause anxiety. People may think seriously about changing their behavior in order to avoid HIV. A good counseling session before the test can give a person important knowledge and tools that he will need to be safe. For example, if someone drinks alcohol, gets drunk, and then has unsafe sex with different partners, you can help her understand the link between alcohol and unsafe sex. The pre-test session is very important; some people will not come back for their test result, and this may be your only chance to talk with them.

If an HIV test is positive, then the person must face new decisions. You can help people tell their sexual partners and their family, and you can help them get health care. When people find out that they have HIV, they will probably want to know about the symptoms of AIDS (see Chapter 2). Some people whose tests are positive may be so shocked that they do not hear or understand what you say. Ask them to come back later to continue talking.

What it means to have HIV

If a person has HIV, it means

1. HIV is in her body, even though she may not be sick or have AIDS.
2. She may pass the virus to others, including babies she may have in the future.
3. She should never donate blood.
4. She may stay healthy for a long time, especially if she takes good care of herself.
5. She needs advice and follow-up counseling.

If an HIV test is negative, it is still important to counsel the person after the test. A negative test does not mean that a person is immune to HIV; the person can still get it later. Talk to the person about the effectiveness of the test and how to prevent HIV infection in the future. A negative test result can give a person hope and a new view of life; if a person took risks in the past, it can help change that behavior.

HIV testing and pregnancy

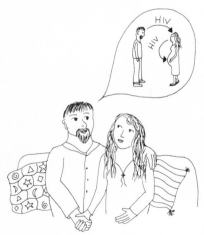

If a man and woman are thinking of having a child, they should talk with each other about the risks of giving HIV to their baby. A man with HIV can pass the virus to his partner, who can in turn pass it to their baby. Pregnant women with HIV should know that pregnancy can make HIV disease worse.

Many times a woman will already be pregnant when she finds out she has HIV.

In some places, drugs that prevent the spread of HIV from mothers to babies will be available (see "Medicines that work against HIV" on page 185). The laws and feelings in her community about abortion and HIV may also play a part in her decision about her pregnancy. Some people feel that having an abortion is not ethical. Families may pressure women to have children at any cost. Other people feel that having children when you have HIV is not moral or responsible. Issues surrounding HIV and women are complex, and people being tested will need support (see Chapter 8).

Answering Jean-Patrice's questions

"Can I get tested for AIDS? How good is the test? If I am negative, does that mean I am immune?"

Jean-Patrice is worried about whether he has AIDS. He is also worried about giving HIV to his girlfriend in his home village. He has other girlfriends in Cayenne and does not know if they have the virus. You can explain to him that he can be tested for HIV. Most people who have AIDS are very ill; usually a test is not necessary to know that they have the disease. The HIV test can be useful, however, for finding out if someone who does not seem ill has HIV.

The HIV test looks for HIV antibodies. Sometimes it takes up to three months for a person's body to make HIV antibodies. If Jean-Patrice has a negative HIV test, there is a small chance that he may still have the virus; he should get tested again in three months. A negative test does not mean that Jean-Patrice is immune to HIV. He can still get the virus from one of his girl-friends if she has HIV. Jean-Patrice should protect himself and his girlfriends by having safe sex.

8

Counseling people about HIV testing

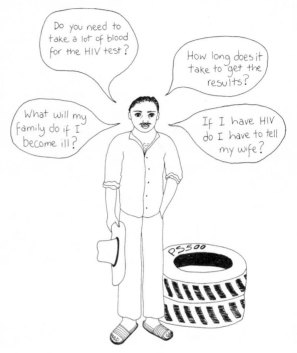

José's story

Assessing HIV risk

Counseling before the test

Waiting for results

Counseling after the test

Answering José's questions

José's story

José is a truck driver in Mexico. He is married and has six children. He works long hours driving his truck from his home in Uruapan to Mexico City. When he is in Mexico City he often has sex with women and men there. A truck driver friend of his is now sick with diarrhea and a cough and has been asked to leave his job. José has become worried that it is because of AIDS. He thinks he might have HIV too and is afraid he may have to tell his wife about his having sex with other people. José wanted to be tested for HIV months ago but did not know where to go. He recently saw a sign for your HIV outreach program, which comes to a truck stop on his route every Friday. This afternoon José comes to visit you and learn about the test. He asks, "Do you need to take a lot of blood for the HIV test? How long does it take to get the result? If I have HIV, do I have to tell my wife? What will my family do if I become ill?"

Assessing HIV risk

Each person has a different risk of having HIV. Talking about a person's risk will help her decide whether to take the test. More importantly, it will give her ideas about how to lower her chance of getting HIV in the future. In areas of the world where many people already have HIV, most people are probably at risk, and it can be difficult to know whose risk is highest and who should be tested. In these areas, for example, nearly everyone who has had sex is at high risk of having been infected with HIV. However, some behavior puts people at

---

Who should be offered an HIV test?

Not everyone who wants an HIV test should have one. People may worry about HIV and ask to be tested even though they are not at risk. By asking some questions, you can find out whether a person is at risk and should be tested. There are three things that it is important to talk about with each person: sexual history, drug use, and whether or not the person has ever had a blood transfusion. You may want to ask some of the following questions, adapting them to your particular area and situation.

1. Why do you think you might have HIV?
2. Have you ever had sex? If so:

   What type of sex have you had—vaginal, oral, or anal? (HIV is more likely to be spread by anal than vaginal sex; it is least likely to be spread by oral sex. See Chapter 5.)

   Have you had sex with someone you know has HIV?

   Have you had sex with anyone you think could have HIV? For example, with a sex worker, with a man who has had sex with other men, with someone who has had a blood transfusion, or with someone from an area with a high rate of HIV infection?

   How many sexual partners have you had in the last year?

   How many sexual partners have you had in your lifetime?

   Do you use condoms during sex? All the time or sometimes?
3. Have you had any sexually transmitted diseases such as syphilis or gonorrhea?
4. Have you ever been given a blood transfusion?
5. Have you ever been given a shot with a needle that had been used on another person without being cleaned afterward?
6. Have you ever been stuck by a dirty needle or medical instrument?
7. Have you ever injected illegal drugs? If so, have you ever shared needles?
8. Have you ever had herpes zoster (also called shingles) or tuberculosis?

If the person answers "yes" to any of these questions, she should probably get tested for HIV.

---

higher risk even in these areas. This behavior includes visiting sex workers, having many sexual partners, having sex with someone who is known to have HIV, and having had other STDs.

Counseling before the test

The HIV test provides a special opportunity for counseling. Sometimes it is the only chance to speak to people in depth about the ways HIV is spread. Because it can be hard to decide to take the test, people are often ready to think about changing behavior that puts them at risk. Offering testing will attract people to your other HIV services, such as treatment for sexually transmitted diseases, family planning, or social services.

Before people are tested for HIV, you can have them develop a plan of action for after they get the test result, whether it is positive or negative. What will they do? Who will they tell? How will they bring it up? What parts of their life will they change? If they have HIV, how will they avoid spreading the virus to other people? You can discuss with them who should take the test, how the test works, and how to avoid HIV. Additional counseling should be done after the test.

It can be helpful to counsel couples together, both before and after the test. This encourages both members to talk about HIV and what they will do with the test results. Sometimes pre-test counseling sessions are done in groups to save time. Although this can be useful, people may be less likely to bring up personal questions in a group than if they are counseled alone or with their partner.

Introductions are important to set the tone for the session. A simple, open-ended question, such as "What brings you here?" or "How can I help you today?" shows you are ready to listen. Later, you can ask more specific questions that will help you understand a person's knowledge of HIV and AIDS. Listen carefully to a person's concerns and questions. Use the time to get a sense of her background and needs.

Next you can discuss basic facts about HIV. Ask each person what he knows about HIV: "How do people get HIV? How can people avoid HIV? Why do people get sick from HIV?" This way, time is not wasted teaching something a person already knows. This also gives you a chance to teach new facts about HIV. Afterward, ask the person to repeat what he has learned; this will help you know if he understood what you were saying. Ask frequently if he has any other questions and listen for an answer. Silence is fine; it often helps bring out important questions or feelings. Sometimes a person's biggest concern is brought up at the end of a meeting.

Explain to people that only a small amount of blood is needed for the test, just one teaspoon (five milliliters) or less for a finger stick test. The body is able to make this amount of blood very quickly, so a person being tested should not feel tired or weak after the blood is taken.

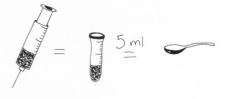

Amount of blood needed for HIV test

Let people know how long they will have to wait for their test results. If they need to wait a few days or a week or two, make a follow-up appointment. Do not use the mail or telephone (where available) for giving test results. By coming to the clinic, people can hear about their test result in a supportive environment where their questions can be answered. They can also receive information about services available to them if they have HIV. Appointments should be made in the same way for people who have positive and negative results. For example, do not schedule people whose results are negative to come in for a five-minute appointment and people whose results are positive to come in for a 30-minute appointment. Rumors can spread about what the length of an appointment means and people may not return for their test results.

Privacy

People may be treated unfairly when it is learned that they have HIV or AIDS. Because of this, information about HIV should be kept in strict confidence. When possible, medical records should be locked in a safe place where only health workers can read them. Counseling should be done in an area where you cannot be overheard. You should consider limiting what is written in a person's records about HIV or diseases specific to AIDS. This helps avoid having information about someone spread to people who do not need to know it and who might discriminate against the person.

People should be told whether their test results will be confidential or anonymous, and what that means (see Chapter 7). How the information is kept may affect whether someone decides to take the test or not.

The meaning of the test

Before the test, explain the meaning of each possible test result. This will help avoid confusion later, when you tell a person the result of his own test.

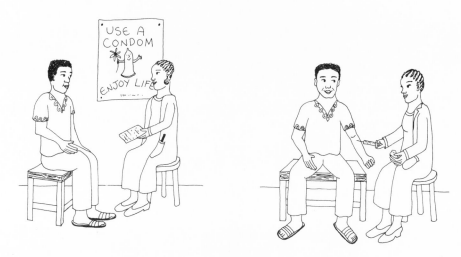

Explain what different test results mean before drawing blood.

A positive test result means that a person has HIV. He could have been infected at any time in the past when he took part in risky behavior—even years earlier. A child may have been infected at birth. A negative test result means that a person does not have HIV. Very rarely, a person with a negative HIV test may still have HIV, because it takes 3 weeks from infection for a person to develop enough antibodies to make the test positive. The person may want to take another test in a month, especially if he or she has recently engaged in any risky behavior.

Waiting for results

Usually people have a lot to think about before getting their test results. They may need to wait as little as an hour or as much as two weeks, depending on the type of test used. The wait usually seems long, whether it actually is or not. While waiting (and worrying), people may think seriously about how they act and how they can change their behavior or living situation to avoid getting HIV in the future. They may think about how they can avoid infecting others if the test turns out to be positive. This is one reason why it is better to do most of the teaching and talking before the test, saving the post-test session for dealing with a person's response to the results. Often when people get their results, they are so nervous or dazed that they are unable to learn new information.

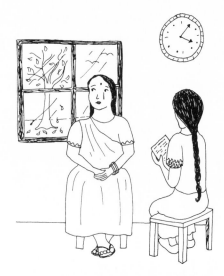

Right after hearing their test results, people may not listen to counseling.

Counseling after the test

Imagine for a moment that after a two-week wait you are on your way to the clinic to hear your HIV test result. You hope to see the familiar face of your counselor. Maybe you will sit in the same chair you sat in two weeks ago. You are nervous as you open the clinic door. What are you thinking at this moment? Do you wonder what your test result is? Do you wonder who will tell you the result? Do you wonder how the news will change your life? Do you wonder if it would be better not to know?

The counseling appointment after the test gives a supportive setting for hearing the news. If the test is negative it gives a person time to ask questions and think about ways to lower their risk of getting HIV in the future. If the test is positive the person will have a chance to talk with someone who knows about HIV and can help them with the bad news.

Counseling people with positive test results

It is hard to give someone news of a positive test. It is difficult to tell someone bad news. However, most people with positive results already guessed that they had HIV; a positive test may be less of a surprise than you think. Fortunately, you will probably give more negative results than positive ones. Prepare beforehand for telling someone a test result; this will make the experience better for you and for the person who took the test. You can do this by thinking carefully about what you are going to say and what the person's responses might be.

Breaking the news

Ask a person what she has been thinking about since taking the test. Find out what worries or questions she has. Arrange for enough time to talk about the issues she raises. When you give the result, use a neutral tone of voice. You might simply say, "Your HIV test was positive," and then wait for the person to respond. A neutral tone and a moment of silence allow someone to feel her own feelings rather than respond to yours. People have many different responses to both positive and negative results. For this reason, let each person set the tone and pace of the discussion according to her own needs.

First reaction

The first feelings that people have after finding out they have HIV may include denial, anger, fear, sadness, hopelessness, and guilt. Most people will be upset, and some may talk about hurting themselves or other people. Help avoid a crisis. Be supportive. Let them know that strong emotions are understandable, but that they should not give up hope. Acknowledge feelings by using simple statements such as "This is probably a scary time for you."

Sometimes people will not accept the results of a positive test. They will insist that they are negative and that there has been a mistake. Do not argue with them. Tell them that the test is almost never wrong but you are willing to discuss the possibility of a second test. People who deny the truth are often the most in need of support; ask them to return for another meeting.

While you should not deny people's worries, it is helpful to talk about things positively. For example, many people believe that having HIV means they will die very soon. Talk about how long it usually takes to become ill. Some people have lived for over fifteen years with the virus. Teaching people ways to stay healthy will build feelings of strength at a time when they may feel powerless. Research is being done that may lead to new treatments for HIV and AIDS.

If you know the person you are counseling, you might talk about difficult times in the past that he handled well. Try to help the person overcome harmful thoughts and focus on solving problems. Help people plan for the future. Talk about the plans they made during the pre-test counseling session. This will remind them that they will not die tomorrow, and it can help change feelings of fear or hopelessness into feelings of strength. Help people find a health worker who knows about treating people with HIV—maybe you!

People will want to talk about their health, their relationships with friends and family, and how to have safer sex to protect sexual partners. By talking openly about these things you will help people accept the fact that their lives are changing. People with HIV should practice safer sex, not only for their sexual partners' protection, but also for their own. Having unsafe sex puts a person at risk of getting sexually transmitted diseases, many of which are more severe in persons with HIV. Additionally, exchanging body fluids with another person who has HIV may make a person sicker, because one person's virus may be more dangerous than another's.

Telling other people

A person with HIV will think about whether to tell other people that she has the virus. The information will affect her relationships with sexual partners, friends, family, employers, and health care providers. More and more people are being taught about HIV and AIDS, but there is still a lot of misunderstanding and fear of the disease. Each person should be warned of the risks and benefits of telling people she has HIV. The goal is to gain support from friends and family while decreasing the risk of discrimination.

People with HIV should start by telling those people who will be the most supportive and those who may also be at risk of having the virus. Everyone with HIV should be strongly urged to tell past and present sexual partners about having HIV. Sexual partners need to know so that they can be tested and can protect *their* partners from infection. When counseling a person with HIV, you should ask him about his sexual partners and how he plans to tell them. Role playing is a useful way to help a person with HIV practice how to tell others (see Chapter 11).

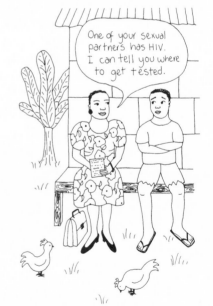

If the person with HIV can tell her partners, this keeps her sexual partners' names confidential. However, some people are reluctant to tell their partners. This can be especially true for women who fear being yelled at, beaten, or thrown out of the house by their partners. In such cases, the person with HIV may ask a health worker to tell the partners that they might have HIV. The name of the person with HIV can be kept confidential or the couple can be counseled together. The health worker can teach the partners about HIV and AIDS and encourage them to be tested.

The following list describes some emotions families or friends may feel when someone they care about tells them that he has HIV. Health workers can talk about some of these possible reactions with people who have a positive test. It will help them prepare for difficult situations. If the health worker has HIV herself, talking about some of her personal experiences can be especially helpful.

Shock. Family members may be shocked and ask, "Why us?" They may be surprised to find out about the situation that put their loved one at risk; for example, a husband or wife may not have known that the other was having sex outside the marriage.

Anger. Families and sexual partners may be angry with a person who has HIV. They may feel betrayed if the person had sex outside the relationship, or they may feel abandoned because the person they love will become ill. The anger may get worse as the person with HIV becomes ill and health workers do not have much medical help to offer. The family or partner may become frustrated. Try to help them understand some of the reasons they might be angry, and let them know that it is natural to be frustrated in the face of these issues.

Fear of infection. Family members and sexual partners may think that they gave HIV to their loved one, or they may worry that their loved one will infect them in the future. It is important to talk with family members about how the virus is and is not spread. HIV is not spread by casual contact, so they do not have to worry about living with someone with HIV or being friends with him, but they should think about changing their sexual behavior to lower the chance that the virus will spread. Sexual partners should think about being tested for HIV themselves.

Fear of being alone. Families and friends may worry about being left alone or isolated from the rest of the community. A serious illness often causes the community to withdraw. Health workers can offer support and let families and friends know that they are not alone. If there are support groups in the community for families and friends of people with HIV, tell people about them.

Guilt. People who are close to others with HIV but don't have the virus themselves may feel guilty about the fact that they do not have the virus. Some people react to this by taking more risks because they care less about their own lives. Other people may think that they or someone in their family did bad things in the past, and that their gods or spirits are now punishing them by giving them HIV.

Shame. Some families or friends may feel ashamed that a person has HIV. They may think that HIV brings dishonor to the family. Families may have less contact with the community because they fear rejection. Explain that no one should feel ashamed to have someone with HIV in the family.

Helplessness. Family and friends may feel helpless in the face of disease. Learning more about HIV and volunteering for an HIV organization can give them a sense that they can help other people and help slow the spread of HIV and AIDS.

The next step

Hearing about positive HIV test results can bring up many strong feelings; a person may not be able to concentrate and may not hear what you are saying. Try to give written information to each person who is able to read, so that she can later read about what she did not hear or understand in your post-test counseling session. Make an appointment for her to come back so that you can talk about health services, support groups for people with HIV, crisis counseling services, and programs for people who use drugs or alcohol.

Counseling people with negative results

A complete counseling session is also important for people who have a negative HIV test. Counseling a person with a negative result is, in many ways, like counseling someone who is positive. The session can start with general questions about what the person has thought about since the last visit. Ask if he has any questions before you tell him the result. After giving the result, give him time to respond with his own feelings and thoughts.

If a person has a negative result, remind him that a negative test only means he does not have HIV now. He can still get HIV in the future.

Most people will feel relieved to receive a negative test result. Sometimes, however, people feel sad or guilty, especially if they have lost friends or loved ones to AIDS.

Sometimes people do not believe that they are negative. They know that they had sex with someone who has HIV and they think that HIV is spread every time a person with HIV has sex. You can tell them that this is not true. In any case, this is the time for a person to develop a strong commitment to staying HIV negative.

Counseling people with indeterminate results

An indeterminate HIV test result is confusing. It means that a person is newly infected and has just begun to make HIV antibodies, or that something else in his blood causes a partially positive test by mistake. Suggest that he take another test in a month. He should practice safe behavior while waiting for the next test.

Ask, "How have you been since the test? What have you thought about? Do you have any questions?"

Give test result in a neutral tone: "Your test is positive/negative/indeterminate."

Wait for a response.

Talk about the following:

    the meaning of the test result

    telling others

    being safe

    staying healthy

    anticipating problems

Review plan made during pre-test session.

For people with a positive test, hand out written information and schedule a follow-up appointment.

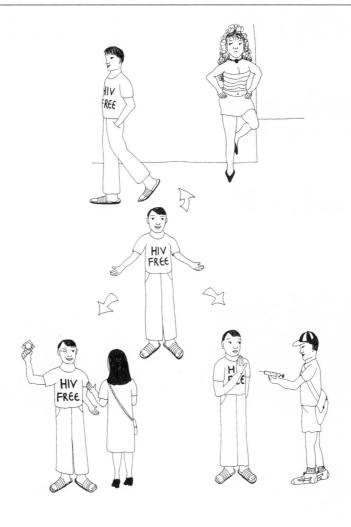

Answering José's questions

"Do you need to take a lot of blood for the HIV test? How long does it take to get the result? If I have HIV, do I have to tell my wife? What will my family do?"

After talking with José, you know there is a chance that he has HIV because he has had unsafe sex with different people. You recommend that he be tested for HIV. Only a little blood is needed, usually about 5 milliliters, or one spoonful. It usually takes between an hour and two weeks to get the result (this depends on the laboratory).

Counseling before and after the test will be helpful whether José has HIV or not. Encourage him to acknowledge his feelings by using simple statements such as "This is probably a difficult time for you." Let him know before taking the test that he should talk with his wife after receiving the results. A positive result may affect his and his wife's decision about having more children. If his wife also has HIV, she could pass the virus on to her baby. If she does not have HIV, she may become infected while trying to become pregnant. If José gets sick, it would be harder for his wife to support another child.

If José's test is positive, he should tell all his other sexual partners as well. They should also be tested. This will help them plan for the future and get early medical care. This is also a chance for you to talk about safer sex at a time when José is likely to listen to you.

José is worried about how his family will survive if he has HIV. These worries often stop people from being tested—they think, "What I do not know will not hurt me." Discuss how knowing whether he has HIV will help José and his family plan for the future. Help him plan for the future, whether his test result is positive or negative.

9

Social and cultural factors that affect the spread of HIV

Odette's story

Odette is a 35-year-old Munukutuba-speaking woman with four children living in Port-Gentil, Gabon. She is a refugee from the neighboring country of Congo. She sells tomatoes and other vegetables in the market but does not have enough money to send her children to school. Her husband of many years was unable to find work for a long time and began to drink too much alcohol. He recently went away to work in the swamps, looking for oil. Although her husband is not around much, Odette has been faithful to him, but she wonders if he has had other sexual partners. She lives with her husband's family, while her own lives in another town.

Odette is worried because her youngest son has had diarrhea for a month. Today she walks into the health clinic in search of treatment for her baby. There is no Munukutuba-speaking counselor, but Odette understands some of your language. She says that she has been feeling tired and wonders if she is pregnant. Yesterday she heard a song about AIDS and children on the radio and it made her worried about her baby. "What should I do about my son's diarrhea?" she asks. "My mother-in-law does not want me in her house. Could she have caused my baby to have AIDS to make us leave?"

Prejudice and discrimination

Social forces such as discrimination and poverty affect who gets HIV and what kind of treatment they get when they become ill. Some people would rather think that only "bad" people get HIV, because if they themselves are "good," then they will not be infected. Of course, this is not true. People and governments need to accept that HIV is everyone's problem and work together to stop the spread of the disease.

Use the facts

HIV is frightening, and people often make decisions based on fear and not facts. This can be seen in many areas of society: government ministers decide to have students from only certain countries tested for HIV, health care workers refuse to care for people with HIV, children are not allowed to go to school if they have HIV, people refuse to buy houses from people with AIDS, and people are fired from their jobs because of people's fears about infection. Actions like these come from emotions; they do not stop the spread of HIV. Make your decisions based on facts, not fear!

Preventing discrimination

All over the world, people with HIV have faced discrimination. Here are some examples of how people have tried to stop this from occurring.

In 1997, Zimbabwe's government established a national code of practice that makes it illegal to discriminate against people with HIV or AIDS.

In Kampala, Uganda, some business owners ask people who are looking for work to take an HIV test. They also hire older workers, who are less likely to have HIV or become infected with it. AIDS activists are trying to keep employers from using HIV tests to decide who to hire. The government is also against required testing, except for people going into the army and those being hired for foreign training.

The southern region of Russia was the first area of the country to be affected by HIV. The virus spread when a child with HIV was hospitalized in Kalmykia province and doctors reused dirty needles that had been used on the child. People with HIV began to experience discrimination. To try to prevent this, the state government passed laws to make sure people with HIV would have free medical care, education, jobs, and better housing.

All people have some type of prejudice—that is, low regard for certain groups of people. Prejudice is often based on how we feel about others' wealth, poverty, sex, ethnicity, political beliefs, or sexual practices. Some peo-

The surgeon and the car accident

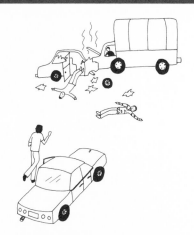

One hot day in July, Philippe was on his way from Yaoundé to Douala in Cameroon. Trucks drive by each other at very high speeds on this road and there are many accidents. Philippe was driving his uncle's car with a trunk full of cloth for his sister's wedding. He drove carefully because he knew of the road's dangers and he was not in a hurry. When he had almost reached Douala, he came upon a terrible accident. A truck filled with many people had collided with a brand-new Mercedes-Benz. The Benz was crushed and a man and his son were thrown from the car. Philippe quickly picked up the injured passengers and drove them to a local hospital. The surgeon was called, saw the young boy, and immediately exclaimed, "That's my son!"

How is this possible?

The surgeon was a woman! (Did you assume that the surgeon was a man?)

ple react negatively to those outside their social, ethnic, racial, or religious group. They believe untrue things about particular groups of people—such as that all skinny people are thieves. You need to be especially aware of your own prejudices, or biases, because they can get in the way of counseling work. Prejudice can prevent counselors from getting to know people and helping them.

The good news is that biases can be unlearned. No one is born with feelings that make them judge people they do not know; people are taught prejudice by others. The first step in freeing oneself from prejudice is to recognize it. In this chapter we describe factors like poverty and discrimination, and we discuss ways to become more understanding of all people with HIV.

Cultural and religious beliefs

People have many ways of explaining health and illness. Some people believe AIDS is caused by a virus. Others believe that AIDS is a punishment for wrongdoing, is caused by bad spirits, or is a result of jealousy.

Find out what people in your community believe about AIDS. Ask each person you counsel what she knows about AIDS. Knowing her ideas will help you build a better counseling relationship. For example, you want to tell someone that condoms can stop HIV. You know that AIDS is caused by a virus. But what if the person thinks that AIDS is caused by magic? It would be difficult for her to understand why condoms will help. Knowing a person's beliefs will tell you where to start your discussion.

Not only do people have different ideas about the cause of AIDS, but they also have different beliefs about how to cure the disease. Often, folk remedies and traditional methods are as good as or better than Western medicine. Other times, though, they may be harmful. Ask about a person's healing beliefs; if they are harmful, carefully challenge them. For example, Odette blames her son's risk of AIDS on her mother-in-law's anger, but the real threat to Odette is more likely her husband's drinking and sexual practices. If a person's beliefs are helpful, say so. No matter how different from yours, treat other people's

Ideas about how HIV is spread can lead people to do strange things. The following story is about a false but common belief about how HIV is spread.

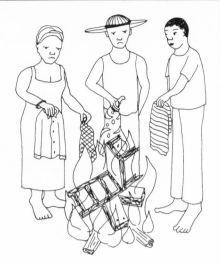

Dominique is a reporter for a newspaper in Guadeloupe. One beautiful sunny day she was driving along the beach to interview a fisherman. The fisherman had caught a marlin that was larger than his boat and everyone on the island was talking about it. Dominique had her camera in her lap, ready to take a picture of the huge fish for her newspaper. Suddenly she saw a small fire off the road in the forest. She pulled over. She approached the flames and saw a group of people standing around. The flames came from a big pile of clothes, furniture, and a bed. She asked why the villagers were burning all these useful things, and they answered that the man who owned the clothes and furniture had died of AIDS.

Dominique was surprised because she knew that clothes do not spread AIDS. At first she thought that the people did not know how HIV is spread because they were from a small village. But later, she asked 50 people in her own town if HIV and AIDS could be spread by clothing or furniture, and was surprised to find out that almost all of the people thought that clothes could spread HIV. Dominique then wrote a story for the newspaper explaining that this belief was untrue and titled it "Clothes do not infect the man!"

beliefs seriously and with respect. Otherwise, they are likely to ignore your suggestions and never come back for more treatment or counseling.

Social and economic status

A person's social or economic position can affect his views about how HIV is spread. It can also change his chance of infection and determine what kind of medical care he gets. For example, an educated person may have learned more about how to avoid HIV. On the other hand, a person with a lot of money may be able to travel to large cities or other countries, which, if he engages in risky behavior there, may increase his chances of getting HIV. In some countries,

In 1997, Nkandu Luo, Zambia's deputy health minister, said that skills training and campaigns to fight poverty should be an important part of anti-AIDS efforts. "Even if people have the best information on AIDS, but they don't have food to eat or they are not involved in anything to bring them income, then we are not going to succeed in our efforts to prevent AIDS."

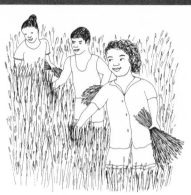

men with a lot of money are more easily able to have several sexual partners than men with little money; again, this can increase the chance of getting HIV. On the other hand, people with less money have more difficulty getting health care, information about HIV, and condoms. People with less money are often forced to travel long distances to find work. They may live in large cities, away from their families and community support. Sometimes they need to exchange sex for food, housing, money, or drugs. It is difficult to avoid HIV under these conditions.

A number of factors can make life especially difficult for women. Having children may force a woman to spend long hours feeding, raising, and caring for them. Childbearing itself, especially in the case of a difficult pregnancy,

Ali and Dunia

Ali is a student at a small college in Alexandria, Egypt. He is studying mathematics and wants to become a schoolteacher. Because his home is up the Nile River in Luxor, Ali lives in a dormitory at the college. Ali's friend Dunia lives in a nearby dormitory. Dunia grew up in Jordan. Both of Dunia's parents were killed in a traffic accident two years ago. She is studying accounting so that she can work for one of the American oil companies in Cairo.

Ali is worried about Dunia because lately she has not been her usual happy self. He asks her what is wrong. She explains that she is having problems with her boyfriend. She is hurt because he has other girlfriends. She is worried about getting pregnant and getting AIDS but does not know how to talk about this with her boyfriend. He has left her many times but he always comes back. Because Dunia is very poor, her boyfriend pays for her food. She needs the food and usually does whatever he wants in return. Ali is frustrated because he knows Dunia may become pregnant or get HIV.

How would you counsel Dunia?

can limit a woman's ability to work. Also, in many countries women do most of the housework and farming. They may also be responsible for caring for elderly family members. This leaves women with less time for education or work outside the home, and it increases their dependence on their husbands and families. In general, women have less money than men. In many parts of the world, this means women have less power in a relationship—less power to ask for safer sex or to make decisions about family planning (that is, about whether to

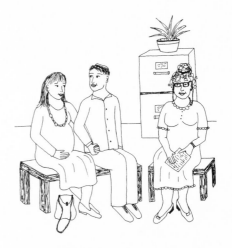

Sometimes it can help to bring your partner with you to HIV counseling.

have children, and if so, how many to have and when to have them). Finally, traditional ideas about women's roles in society may make it difficult for women to talk about sex. When women are counseled by other women they may talk more openly than when counseled by a man. Some women may feel freer to speak their mind when their partner is not present. Other women may want their partner to be present because the partner may treat information more seriously when it comes from you than from them.

Most societies want women to have only one sexual partner. In contrast, in many places men are encouraged to have more than one partner. This can be dangerous for them and for their partners. A man who has sex with women outside his partnership or marriage may feel ashamed and may not tell his wife or girlfriend. This puts the woman at risk.

Ethnicity

Ethnicity refers to a person's cultural group or tribe. Often, one ethnic group controls money and resources and denies other groups an equal share. Members of some ethnic groups may be forced from their homes, prevented from having certain jobs, restricted from particular schools, or physically attacked. In many parts of the world, ethnic groups are waging war against each other.

Counseling people from different ethnic groups is challenging. Sometimes groups speak different languages and have different beliefs about health and illness. Try to have people from different ethnic groups work with you; that way people can be counseled by someone more familiar with their group.

Indigenous (native) people in many countries are at a higher risk of getting HIV than other people. This is mostly because indigenous people are more likely to suffer from discrimination, live in poverty, and have less access to education and health care.

For example, HIV infection is growing among Brazil's native tribes. Many of the tribes are poor, and some of their people have had to move to larger cities to find work. In the cities, they are exposed to HIV. In 1997, the government started an AIDS awareness program with the tribes. Much more needs to be done.

In 1997, the rate of HIV infection in Australia was dropping. However, HIV infection among indigenous peoples—including Aborigines and Torres Strait Islanders—was increasing. Educational programs were begun to talk with people about sexual health, HIV, and other sexually transmitted diseases.

Making an effort to understand more about the cultural groups you counsel will make other people more comfortable and open to your suggestions.

Discussions about HIV are sensitive and complex. Make sure people understand the language you are using. Try to have a counselor who speaks the person's native language. If this is not possible, you can use an interpreter. Unfortunately, having a third person in the room can make it harder for people to talk about personal issues. If an interpreter is embarrassed, she may change a person's story. She may not understand all the questions or answers. But it is better to use an interpreter than not to be able to speak with someone at all.

Education

Education changes how people see themselves. It also affects a person's health. Often, the more educated a mother is, the healthier she is because she knows how to take care of herself. The healthier a mother is, the healthier her child will be. The level of a person's education can help or hurt your efforts to counsel someone. For example, a person who is able to read may have read newspapers and billboards about AIDS. He may already know something about HIV. You could teach him using written materials. The ability to read and write may mean that a person feels comfortable learning in a school setting.

A person who does not read or write relies on other sources of information, such as radio, television, and friends. She often thinks more in terms of real-life situations. In this case, telling stories about other people with AIDS may teach more than listing facts about the number of people in the country with HIV. Using visual aids such as posters, drawings, and videos can be especially helpful. People who cannot read often learn better from their own experience than from information given in a student-and-teacher setting. When counseling such a person, it is also better to ask more concrete (exact) questions; for example, ask "When you last had sex, did you use a condom?" rather than "Should condoms always be used for sex?"

Written materials such as pamphlets can help with your counseling. People may have questions after you have spoken with them, and the written information can help answer these. It can also remind people of facts they have forgotten. They can share the pamphlet with others. People who have difficulty reading can still be given written materials; their friends or family can read the materials to them.

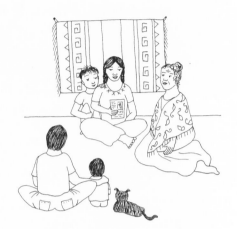

Counseling checklist

Ask yourself these questions while counseling:

What does this person already know about AIDS? At what level should I start the session?

What languages does this person speak? Should I get an interpreter?

Can this person read? Has he gone to school? Do I have any information sheets to give him?

Is this person understanding me?

Sexual practices

Health counselors often have little training in human sexuality and rely mostly on their own experience. This means they often do not feel comfortable talking about sexual practices. Some counselors are prejudiced against certain sexual practices. You can overcome your own prejudices by creating a broader sense of what is normal. For example, if you have a difficult time talking about anal sex and HIV, then talk about it with coworkers. This will help you feel more comfortable talking about sex and HIV while counseling. A good counselor should be able to talk about most issues comfortably.

Try to be neutral when discussing sexual practices. It is important not to judge people if you want to have an open discussion with them. Avoid using labels or names; instead, talk about specific practices. For example, ask a man "Have you ever had sex with a man?" instead of "Are you gay?" A man who has had sex with men would answer yes, even if he did not consider himself gay (homosexual). You would then be able to talk with him about reducing his risk of getting HIV. The more comfortable you are talking about sex, the more comfortable people around you will be when they talk about sex.

Using neutral language	
When counseling people, be sure to use neutral, not biased, language. Biased language may offend people. Neutral language will help lead to a more open discussion.	
Biased	Neutral
Are you a slut? promiscuous?	How many sexual partners do you have?
Are you a prostitute? hooker? gigolo?	Have you ever traded sex for money, food, or a place to live?
Are you a drunk? wino?	How often do you drink alcohol? About how many drinks a day?
Are you a drug addict? junkie? shooter?	Have you ever used drugs? Which ones?
Are you a homo? fag? fairy?	Have you ever had sex with a man? (to a man)
Are you a dyke? lesbo? diesel?	Have you ever had sex with a woman? (to a woman)

Sex means different things to different people, and its meaning often varies by culture. It can be used to show feelings, have children, provide physical release, gain a sense of closeness or attractiveness, or be a means of getting money or fulfilling an obligation. With an open mind you can develop an understanding with each person that can lead to a free discussion about sex.

Sexual orientation

Certain groups of people may have difficulty getting services such as health care and education. They may be excluded because of their tribe or ethnic

A doctor and his patient

A doctor who practiced for many years in a small town was seeing a patient for the first time. The patient had abdominal pain and was vomiting. The doctor thought that she might be pregnant. He asked her a few questions:

"Are you married?"

"No."

"Are you sexually active?"

"Yes."

"Do you use birth control?"

"No."

"Could you be pregnant?"

"No."

The doctor insisted on doing a pregnancy test on the patient's urine. The test came back negative. When he told her, the woman laughed and explained that there was no way that she could be pregnant because her sexual partner was a woman.

group, their lack of money or resources, their political beliefs, or their "sexual orientation." Sexual orientation refers to whom people are attracted to and have sex with. Heterosexual ("straight") people have sex with people of the opposite sex; homosexual ("gay") people have sex with people of the same sex; bisexual people have sex with both women and men. Gay and bisexual women and men often experience severe discrimination. In the industrialized world HIV has especially affected gay men, and because of this they have experienced even worse discrimination than before the days of AIDS.

Drug and alcohol use

Using drugs or alcohol can increase a person's risk of getting HIV. HIV can be spread if needles are shared during drug use. Drugs and alcohol affect a person's judgment; some people may risk unsafe sex when they are under the influence of one or both. Many types of people inject drugs—mothers, merchants, doctors, street people. Do not assume that someone does not use drugs because that person does not "look" like a drug user.

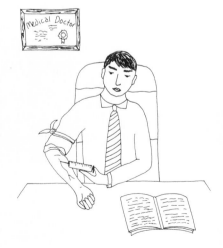

Reaching out to drug users is difficult but not impossible. Some people think that because a person uses drugs she is unwilling or unable to change her behavior. Many drug users *are* self-destructive, but outreach workers have found that many others are interested in changing their behavior once they learn about the dangers of getting HIV. Many drug users know a great deal about the way HIV is spread and have changed their behavior to reduce their risk. You can provide the education and materials to help them change.

Age

Young adults are a special challenge for the HIV worker. Passing from childhood to adulthood is difficult and exciting. In most places, youths depend heavily on friends of the same age for ideas and information. These friends often influence their behavior more strongly than the youths' parents.

Often, young people are not concerned about the future. They may feel immortal and find it hard to believe they could become sick or die. Young people often think, "I can take risks and nothing bad will happen to me." For example, in the United

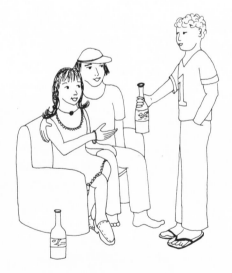

Sometimes young adults listen to each other more than to their elders.

In Zambia and some other parts of Africa, older men think that young women are less likely to have HIV. These men single out young girls for sexual favors. In Zambia this practice is called the "sugar daddy syndrome." Many of the older men already have HIV and spread it to the younger women. The infection rate among young girls is six times as high as the rate among boys the same age.

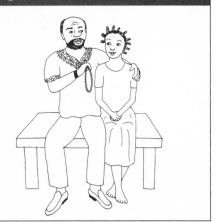

States, they may jump off high rocks into rivers to prove that they are brave. Young people often take risks with sex or drugs; they are curious and want to explore new experiences. They may not think about pregnancy or AIDS.

Written materials are often boring for young people. Theater, music, and video are better ways to reach them (see Chapter 12). Young people may not like authority figures, including health workers. But all of this does not mean that young people do not need your help. Talk about the issues that are important to them as well as those that are important to you. Talk with parents about doing the same. Have young people who already know about HIV talk with other young people. This "peer counseling"—counseling among equals—often allows a more open discussion.

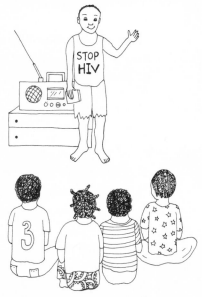

Each person is a part of his community. There are many types of communities. For example, a person's family, village, coworkers, friends, drinking buddies, and schoolmates are all communities. Each of these groups influences how a person thinks and acts. Understanding the different communities in people's lives will help you counsel them about HIV. For example, a teenager may rely on friends for HIV information. His friends may not be worried about HIV and may pressure him to drink and have sex. Another person may be far away from her village. Being far away from home may make her care less about the social rules of her family. For example, being far away from her husband may lead her to have sex with another man. Communities can also be your allies in helping people avoid HIV. If you are teaching a child about HIV, he may share what he learned with his parents. Seeing the individual as part of a "bigger picture" can help you be a better counselor.

Answering Odette's questions

"What should I do about my son's diarrhea? My mother-in-law does not want me in her house. Could she have caused my baby to have AIDS to make us leave?"

Odette is faced with many difficulties. She has asked whether her baby could have AIDS, but she has other worries as well. Odette's situation shows the need for you to see HIV risk as only a part of a person's life. Let us examine the social factors affecting Odette.

1. Economics—Odette is poor.
2. Ethnicity and language—Odette is Munukutuba-speaking. Munukutuba-speaking people have a history of discrimination in some areas. She may not trust you.
3. Belief system—Odette believes that AIDS can be spread by bad will.
4. Knowledge about AIDS—Odette has heard about AIDS but does not know how it is spread.
5. Sexual practices—Odette has had sex only with her husband, but he is away from home much of the time and might have other sexual partners.
6. Alcohol—Odette's husband drinks.
7. Personal health—Odette may be pregnant and may have HIV.
8. Son's health—Odette's baby has diarrhea and might have AIDS.
9. Family support—Odette lives with her husband's family. Her husband's mother does not like her. She is far away from her own family.

The fact that Odette is poor, alone, and has children means that she has a lot of important priorities other than HIV. If she is hungry and is worried about losing her housing, then HIV risk may not seem very important to her. Because she has no money and lives with her husband's family, she may not have any bargaining power for adopting safer sex practices with her husband.

Because Odette is Munukutuba-speaking, she may not have access to information or services. The Munukutuba-speaking people also have certain beliefs about HIV and its spread that should be addressed. Talk with Odette about what she knows about AIDS, and help her learn in areas where she is less knowledgeable.

The fact that her husband drinks and is away from home means that he may have other sexual partners. Ask Odette if she thinks her husband has other sexual partners and if she herself drinks or uses drugs.

Odette thinks she may be pregnant. Ask about her periods and consider asking her to take a pregnancy test. Family planning may be useful. Odette is worried about AIDS. After talking with her more about her chances of having HIV, you may want to offer an HIV test. If Odette is HIV positive, Odette's son may have AIDS. If her son is younger than fifteen months, the standard HIV test will not work; she should bring him back for testing when he is older. However, it is likely that the baby's diarrhea has nothing to do with HIV. The diarrhea may be serious even if it is not caused by HIV, and it should be treated.

You may not entirely understand Odette's situation, but you can encourage her to talk about it. This will allow you to build a relationship with her and answer questions she may have. By listening to her ideas you will learn about her problems, and then together you will be able to develop a plan to reduce her risk for HIV or cope with being infected.

10

How to support and care for a person with HIV

I do not want to live now that I have HIV.

Angela's story

Angela is a young woman who lives in Rio de Janeiro, Brazil. She works at an office downtown and lives with her boyfriend. She and her boyfriend are close to her family, which also lives in the city. Angela is two months pregnant and has felt more tired than usual. She has also had some diarrhea. She came to your clinic for some medicine and had some laboratory tests done, including one for HIV. The HIV test was positive. She does not have the courage to tell her boyfriend about the test. She says to you, "I do not want to live now that I have HIV."

Facing challenges together

Having HIV is isolating. Most people do not know very much about it and are afraid of the virus. Some people think that living near someone with HIV will give them the disease. Friends and family members may abandon someone who has HIV. Coworkers may not want to work with a person who has HIV. Even though HIV cannot be spread in these ways, many people do not know this and avoid contact with anyone who has it.

Supporting people with HIV can be a rewarding experience for a health worker, family member, or friend. The work can also be very demanding. People with HIV need emotional support and physical comfort. People are afraid when they find out they have HIV or AIDS—they fear being left alone, feeling pain, and dying. Having a chronic and fatal disease can be overwhelming. The reaction of the community can make it worse. If you have HIV yourself, you can be a special source of support for others who have the virus. Through your support, you can make a difference in a person's life.

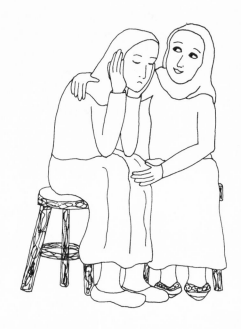

People with HIV must deal not only with medical problems, but also with social and emotional problems. People with AIDS worry about what will happen to their spouses and children when they become ill or after they die. They worry about how they will pay for medical expenses. They feel sad, fearful, angry, and anxious. They may lose hope in the future. These are normal feelings for anyone with a serious illness. These feelings may become so strong that the person cannot carry on with day-to-day activities. When this happens, you can help people find ways to cope with their feelings.

On the other hand, knowing that they have a fatal illness may give people the courage to focus on what is important to them. A serious illness can give people the opportunity to change or walk away from situations that are unpleasant or unhealthy. Many health workers find it rewarding to work with people who are seriously ill because the health worker shares their new sense of purpose. Some people see being infected with HIV as a challenge; they want to be in charge of their household, their finances, and their health. Others may feel less able and need more help. Remind people with HIV that needing and asking for help is normal. Help people with HIV and their families find a balance between dependence and independence.

There are many ways to live with HIV. Some people with HIV do not let others know that they have the virus. Some people become active in fighting the epidemic when they find out they have HIV. Helping someone else avoid the virus provides a sense of purpose. Helping others can give people with HIV a sense of community and self-worth even when their own lives are difficult. Just as people with alcoholism or cancer help others who have the same problems, people with HIV can reach out to others. Many people with HIV talk about AIDS in schools and at community meetings. Some become HIV counselors. Others work as activists for improving services for people with HIV. Some volunteer to be friends or "buddies" for other people with HIV. Each chooses to live with HIV in her own way.

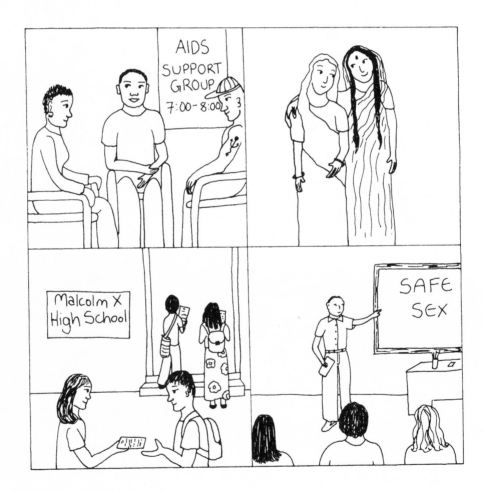

Some people do not believe that HIV is a threat to them. Others think that since they do not belong to a risk group (such as drug users) they will not get the virus. People with HIV have a special ability to reach other people and help them understand how they might be at risk.

In the city of Santa Cruz, California, in the United States, people with HIV help educate other people about AIDS. Six HIV-infected men who were willing to share their personal stories with the community organized Project First Hand. At community meetings, they shared their "firsthand" experiences of living with HIV. By telling their own stories they were able to help people relate to HIV on a personal level. The men were role models for other people with HIV in the community.

Over time, more people with HIV volunteered for the program. They went through short training classes about HIV and public speaking. Then, together they held a small meeting where they practiced talking about their experiences with HIV.

Project First Hand then set up meetings in the community. Health workers were there to help with technical questions and any hostile people in the audience. Friends asked questions if the crowd was too shy or timid. People who have heard the talks have been so moved that they have written letters of support to the speakers. You may want to start such a program in your own community.

Denial and other emotions

Some people do not believe that they have HIV even when a health worker tells them they do. They are not able to face the truth. They do not want to believe that they will die. They do not want to know that a person they love may have given them HIV, or they do not want to think that they may have given the virus to someone they love. Denial can be dangerous for a person with HIV and for others. People who are "in denial" do not take care of themselves because they do not believe that they are sick. If they 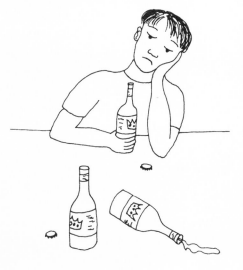 refuse to take precautions, they can give the virus to others. Sometimes people turn to alcohol or drugs in order to forget that they have the virus.

Sometimes people are in denial after hearing that they have had a negative test. They find it hard to believe that they have not been infected, or they do not want to recognize that fact. For example, a woman whose husband has HIV may not want to believe that she had a negative test, because it means she will have to change how she has sex with her husband or leave him.

Yet denial is not all bad. Some denial helps people deal with the day-to-day challenges of life and plan for the future. Denial may help people live without thinking about the seriousness of their illness all of the time.

People with HIV often must cope with many strong emotions. They may have recently lost a loved one to AIDS. Some may feel guilty about the behavior that led to their infection. Most fear rejection from people around them. They may feel that they do not want to continue living, and they may even make plans to kill themselves. You should ask about these feelings and explain that it is normal to have them. You can work with people on ways to cope with these feelings. Anyone who is thinking of killing himself should be taken seriously. Ask him to promise to contact you or someone he trusts before he attempts suicide. Although this may seem silly, it works; just talking with someone often prevents people from harming themselves.

Family counseling

People with HIV have family, friends, and coworkers who will all be affected by their illness. In most communities the family is the basic unit of social organization. Families are able to survive many types of stress. Most families have dealt with death, separation, and economic hardship. HIV and AIDS place new strains on a family. Usually it can adapt, but occasionally a family breaks up when one of its members has HIV. When you sense that this is a possibility, try to help family members get the support they need to stay together. It can be useful to meet with the entire family. Family members may have questions about how to deal with HIV. You can help them talk about problems, solve conflicts, learn how to support each other, and find other sources of help from the community or government.

If a parent has HIV or AIDS, encourage her to talk about it with her children. Children often can tell that something is wrong. They may already have had one parent die of AIDS. It is important for parents to talk with their children about what to expect in the future, even if this might include becoming an orphan.

Help parents plan for their children's future

When adults with HIV die, they often leave behind children. Many parents with HIV worry about this and try to arrange for their children to be cared for by others, but in areas where HIV is widespread this can be difficult. Millions of children have been orphaned by HIV.

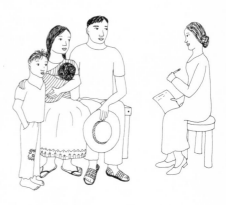

Parents often need support to appoint a guardian or make a will that leaves family assets to wives or children and gives other instructions about the children's future. A counselor can help parents see this planning as security for the family rather than just preparing for death. Caregivers of orphans also need support, especially in places where HIV is very common. This support can be through counseling, parenting training, burial and lending funds, community food programs, shared childcare, or help in paying school fees. Orphans should also be provided HIV counseling and testing so that they can receive care and treatment if needed.

Children not yet orphaned but living with ill and dying parents also need support, to make sure their needs for food, attention, education, and health care are being met.

If a woman has HIV, the chances are that one out of every three babies she gives birth to will have HIV. People with HIV will need help making decisions about family planning. Encourage people with HIV to talk with their partners about family planning. This is a time when giving accurate information and supporting someone with HIV will most help her.

Supporting children with HIV

Children with HIV, even young ones, need to know that they are sick. Younger children may only need to know a little bit about HIV. Give them short, simple answers to their questions. Older children understand more and need correct information and honest answers. If they do not get this information from you or their family, they may get the wrong information from someone else. A child with HIV may suffer silently because of shame or fear. She may have problems sleeping or trouble at school. She may avoid family and friends. Warn families about these signs and help them to talk openly with children who have HIV.

Support groups

It is often useful for a group of people with the same problem to get together and talk about their lives. "Support groups" of people with HIV give people a chance to talk about their problems and successes. People with HIV can learn how to deal with common problems from other people in the group. Support groups help members feel less lonely. People gain strength from their group because they know that they are not alone in struggling with HIV.

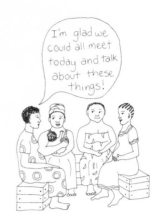

There are different types of support groups. "Drop in" groups meet regularly but people go to meetings only when they want help with a particular problem or when an emergency arises. In other groups, the same people meet weekly for a few months; everyone goes to the meetings, whether or not they have a particular problem to talk about that day. There are also long-term groups that last for years. Long-term groups may be especially useful because they allow people to get to know each other well. These groups also experience the sadness of having members of the group become sick and die.

It is helpful when groups are made up of people with similar lifestyles. The members understand each other's situation and language. You can start support groups that are made up of people with similar backgrounds, such as people of the same social or ethnic background, or people who share a certain risk or condition, such as sex workers, drug users, or pregnant women.

Support groups are also useful for the families and friends of people who have HIV. Even though these people do not have HIV, they may fear losing a friend, becoming infected, or being shunned by their communities and families. A support group can help them with many of the problems they face in having a loved one with HIV.

Care for people with HIV

A person with HIV can live a longer, healthier life with some simple and low cost interventions. Medicines to treat HIV are important (see the appendix at the end of this book), but there are many other measures that can also make a difference in a person's health. See the next page for a sample list of interventions for helping people with HIV.

Cotrimoxazole (trimethoprim/sulfamethoxazole) is a low cost antibiotic that prolongs the lives of children and adults with HIV and prevents malaria and diarrhea, and avoid hospitalization. See the appendix at the end of this book for information on giving this medicine.

Safe drinking water is important for everyone. It is essential for people with HIV because diarrhea caused by unclean water is more common and severe for them. Simple methods for cleaning drinking water are boiling for 3–5 minutes, or adding 5 drops of 5% bleach solution to every liter of water. Also, try pouring water into cups or pots, instead of dipping them back into a full bucket of water, which spreads germs to the water that everyone shares.

Medicine to prevent TB (isoniazid). Tuberculosis (TB) is a common and dangerous lung infection. It is especially common and deadly in people with HIV. Some HIV treatment programs are now giving medicine called isoniazid for 6 to 9 months to prevent TB. Note: it is important *not* to treat people who *already* have TB with isoniazid because people who already have TB need more than one drug. If possible, everyone should be tested for TB before receiving isoniazid, and no one with symptoms of TB (coughing, fever, weight loss, night sweats) should be treated with isoniazid without being tested first. See the section on TB in the appendix for more information about diagnosing and treating TB.

Bed nets treated with insecticides can prevent malaria, a common infection passed by mosquitoes. Problems from malaria are more common and dangerous in people with HIV.

Good nutrition and multivitamins improve the health and prolong the lives of people with HIV, and lower the chances of a mother passing HIV on to her baby. The best way to get vitamins is by eating a variety of nutritious foods like fruits, vegetables, grains, beans, eggs, milk, and meats every day. Taking multivitamin pills every day may offer additional protection.

Offering counseling, testing, and treatment for HIV to family members can help people with HIV talk openly about their status with their partners and family. It can help people with HIV get more support and help from their families, including the support they need to take medicines. It is also useful because many family members of people with HIV are also infected with HIV, but do not know it because they have not been tested. Providing testing, treatment, and a regular supply of condoms to people with HIV and their partners prevents transmission in a couple where one person has HIV and the other does not, and can help prevent transmission from mother to child. Providing testing to family members allows those who have HIV to seek care and treatment.

Social support

All people with HIV will at some time need help. In some countries this will come from their families. In other countries this will come from the community or the government. For example, counseling, home care, needle-exchange programs, and assistance with food, shelter, or transportation may all be available. Find out what services are available and direct people to them when needed. If there are no services available, start some. This may mean starting a support group for people with HIV, making a list of health workers and counselors who work with people with HIV, or setting up a "buddy system" where people with HIV volunteer to be friends to others who are infected. Be creative and talk with people who have HIV about their needs and how they can be met.

Home care

Most families take care of sick members at home. It is often the best way to care for people with HIV. But some people are afraid to care for loved ones with HIV at home. You can help people get over this fear and give practical advice on how to best give home care. With a few precautions, it is possible to care for people with HIV safely at home. You should remind people who are thinking of home care that HIV has never been spread by sharing food, cookware, towels, or other household items.

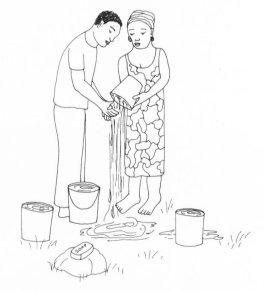

The real risk with home care is for people with HIV. They catch diseases from other people in the household, not the other way around. Even colds or the flu can be serious for someone with AIDS. Some simple things will help people live more happily at home. Living areas

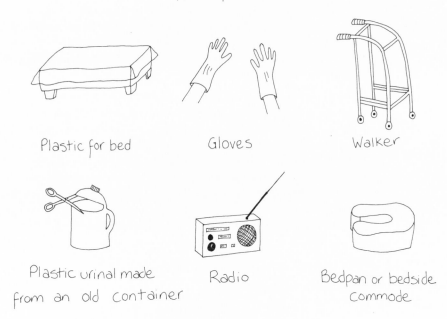

Supplies for home care

Plastic for bed

Gloves

Walker

Plastic urinal made from an old container

Radio

Bedpan or bedside commode

should be clean. Rooms should have plenty of light and air. People with HIV can cook for others without any risk of passing the infection. If they have open sores they should avoid cooking until the sores are better. Anyone who cooks should wash his hands with soap and clean water before preparing food. Dishes should be washed in hot, soapy water. Foods that have dirt on them should be well washed. This is especially true for vegetables grown with animal or human stool as fertilizer. All people should wash their hands with soap after going to the bathroom to prevent the spread of disease.

There are many simple things that can be used to make life at home easier for people with HIV and their families. Some of them may already be in a person's home, such as a radio, a bedpan, gloves, or a walker.

People with HIV have many needs and there are never enough services to help. Money and other resources are often lacking and people with HIV and their families often feel alone in their personal struggle against the disease. You can be a source of hope and help for people and their families.

The AIDS Care and Prevention Programme at the Chikankata Hospital in southern Zambia is a good example of home-based care and prevention efforts in Africa. The program's three-stage effort includes providing medical and nursing care, offering free counseling, and teaching other communities about HIV.

In the home care part of the plan, health care workers make home visits. These visits are made not only for people with HIV and AIDS but for people with serious conditions like epilepsy and cancer. This approach helps avoid discrimination against the people being visited. The home care team teach families about HIV and about practical matters in home care, like how to make a solution (oral rehydration solution) to replace fluids lost by diarrhea. They also draw blood samples and ask families how the team can best help them. Hospitals are often overcrowded and better care can be given at home. These home visits help both the family and the hospital work more effectively.

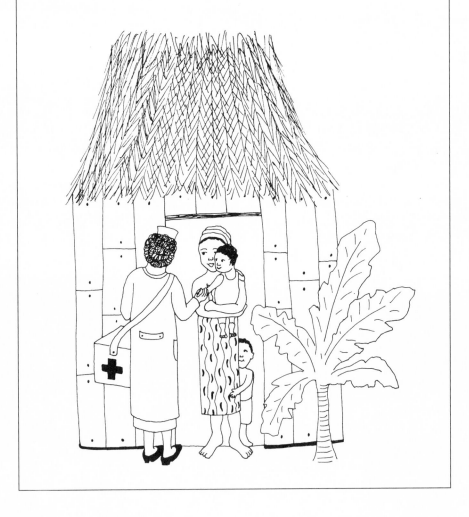

Support for health workers

People who counsel or care for very ill people sometimes become sad and tired. This "burnout" may happen if health workers do not have sufficient time to rest and talk about their own sense of frustration and loss.

Burnout can be emotional, intellectual, physical, or all three. It affects how people do their job. People start to feel tired, helpless, or hopeless. Even workers who usually have a lot of energy and hope may find themselves struggling with burnout. It is important for you to realize that this may occur and to take steps to avoid it.

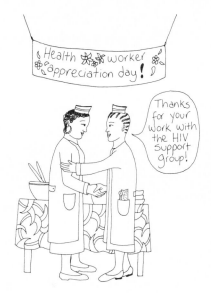

Burnout

Here are some things that can help prevent burnout among health workers.

1. Keep a sense of humor; it helps in stressful situations.
2. Take on a variety of jobs so that you are not doing one stressful job all of the time. This will keep you interested in your work.
3. Make sure you work a reasonable number of hours. Most people who work too much do not work well after a while.
4. Encourage volunteers and reward them with parties or small gifts to let them know their work is appreciated. Make yourself available to answer questions, and acknowledge their efforts in front of others.
5. Recognize work that is well done. People need to know they are doing a good job. Each person needs something different, so give personal compliments.
6. Keep your eyes on the big picture—all the good things in life—so that you do not get lost in the day-to-day struggle.
7. Recruit people who are dedicated and are from the community with which they will be working. They are often more committed and comfortable with the job.
8. Give people days off from their jobs so that they can rest and recover from stress and the strong emotions they may experience at work.
9. Everyone can burn out, even a director or group leader. Be aware of signs of burnout in yourself and others, and work together to avoid it.

How to support Angela

"I do not want to live now that I have AIDS."

Angela is clearly feeling sad and overwhelmed by the news of having HIV. This is understandable, but she has other reasons to be hopeful. She has HIV infection but does not have AIDS. She has a boyfriend who loves her and can help her cope with her illness. She has a family that cares for her. She will live to see the birth of her child. There are medicines that can treat some of the illnesses she will get in the future, and people with HIV are now living longer than they did in the past.

You can talk with Angela about telling her boyfriend about her HIV test. This will bring up many issues, including whether he or she has had sexual partners outside their relationship. It may help for you and Angela to practice how she will tell him that she has HIV. You can offer to talk with her and her boyfriend together about how to live with HIV. There will be many issues you will want to talk about with them, including whether Angela's boyfriend might want to get tested and the fact that the virus can spread from mothers to their babies. Angela may want to talk with other people, especially pregnant women, who have HIV. If there are no support groups in her area, you can help Angela start one. Angela spoke about not wanting to live. Talk about suicide should always be taken seriously. Try to meet with Angela regularly so that she does not feel alone. Encourage her to think positively.

11

Training HIV health workers

How do I stir up interest within the group?

How do I involve everyone?

What if people are too shy to talk?

HIV IS NOT SPREAD BY:

Phan's story

How do we learn?

Who will come to your training session?

Where should you teach?

Getting the session started

Helping others lead

Using language and methods that work

Serving as an example

After the session

Answering Phan's questions

Phan's story

Phan lives in Vietnam. He is a village health worker who recently took part in a training class on HIV in the nearby capital of Hanoi. He went because people in his village were sick with AIDS and a rumor had spread that the virus was in the village water. Phan did not think HIV could be spread by water, but he was not sure. He wanted to find out the truth.

After he returned from the training, Phan realized that his village needed more people who knew about HIV and AIDS. They would be able to teach others and stop false rumors about the virus. A few people offered to help do this. Phan has planned a meeting to speak about what he learned in the training class, but he is nervous about leading a group; he has always been more comfortable talking one-on-one. He wonders, "How do I stir up interest within the group? How do I involve everyone, even the people who usually get bored? What if people are too shy to talk about issues like sex and drug use?"

How do we learn?

The best way to learn something is by doing it. Most people learn to farm by working in the fields, instead of by reading about farming in a book. People can also learn from talking with each other, or reading, or hearing the advice of others. This chapter describes different ways to help people learn. It can be used as a guide for training health workers or teaching in the community. You can adapt the ideas in this chapter to meet the needs of your community.

A health worker's most important task is helping people take control of their health. This is especially true for an HIV health worker because prevention is so important. Training sessions are an important part of this process. The best teachers get people involved and help spark new ideas. They do not confuse people or make them feel stupid for not knowing things or believing things that are not true. Good teachers do not bore people, because when people are bored they will turn away from the chance to learn.

Most of the teaching styles used in formal schooling are based on a teacher telling students what the teacher feels is important to know and then testing them to see if they remember it all. HIV health workers in the Dominican Republic say this is like "pouring water into a sieve instead of a pot." Many times people do not remember information because they were not interested in 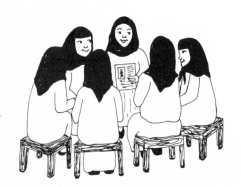 learning it in the first place. Many people have not gone to school and are not used to a one-way flow of facts from "teacher" to "student." It is said that good teaching is drawing ideas out of students, not putting ideas into them. Sharing information in both directions is a better way for a health worker to teach.

Who will come to your training session?

Before you start your training session, think about who will participate. In some areas of the world, almost everyone has friends or family members with HIV. In these areas, many of the people in your training session will have HIV, and the discussions will be different than in areas where few people have personal connections with people who have the virus. Some people will have been inspired by friends or family with HIV to learn more about caring for people who are ill and preventing the spread of the virus. Others may be health workers, sex workers, or community workers active in HIV issues.

Think about having sessions that include people with similar backgrounds. For example, this could mean having one training group for teenagers, another for women, and another for people who have HIV. People have different reasons for becoming interested in learning more about HIV, and you can ask people to talk about some of these during the training sessions. Having groups made up of people with common backgrounds allows people to speak more freely about issues that they might not feel comfortable talking about in a larger group.

Child-to-child teaching

In many places in the world older children care for their younger sisters and brothers while their parents work. Some care for younger brothers and sisters because their parents have died. Few of them have the time to go to school. These children act as parents but often do not know how to care for babies and very young children. Many countries have started programs that work with these children.

Diarrhea is a leading cause of death in children. It can be especially harmful in children with AIDS. In Maharashtra, India, a child-to-child teaching program was started to help teach children about treating and preventing diarrhea. A health worker spends a few hours a day teaching the older children. Often one of the younger children has diarrhea. The health worker uses this as an opportunity to teach about the danger signs of dehydration (when the body loses too much water), how to make oral rehydration fluid, and when to visit a clinic for help. Children can follow the health of a friend with diarrhea as she is being treated. Often the children are inspired when the child gets better and they go home and teach their families what they have learned. You can bring children in your area together and teach them about HIV. They can then go home and teach their sisters, brothers, and parents.

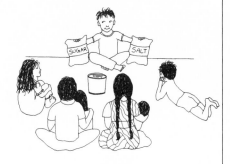

Where should you teach?

Teaching can happen in many places. "Formal" teaching is usually done in a school, clinic, public building, or under a tree. Others teach "informally," while cooking, walking, milking the cows, or weeding the yams. The best place to train people depends on whom you are trying to reach. For example, it may be better to talk with sex workers in the nightclub before they start work. This way they may think about what they learned while they work. Health care workers can be reached at the clinic. Teachers may feel most comfortable learning at school. You can use a barbershop to talk with men in the community. Traditional healers will learn better in their own homes than in a school or clinic. Find people where they live and work; do not make them come to you.

Getting the session started

How you set up your training session makes a difference. Sitting in a circle is a simple way to involve everyone. In a circle everyone can see each other's face. People can share ideas more easily, instead of just being an audience for the teacher. By sitting on the same level as the group, you help people feel comfortable sharing ideas with you.

Later, especially if the group is large, you can split into smaller groups. The groups can then teach each other. Ask each smaller group to teach the larger group the most important things its members learned from each other.

Start the first session by explaining what you are planning for the day. Then ask people to introduce themselves. Self-introductions help people feel more comfortable talking to each other. One way to have people introduce themselves is to have each person explain who she is, why she came to the training session, and what she most wants to learn. Another way to start is to get a ball or a coconut. Have everyone stand in a circle and toss the coconut from one person to another. As each person gets the fruit have him say his name and where he is from and give a word describing himself that begins with the first letter of his name. For example, Kwame could catch the coconut and say, "I am Kwame from Accra, Ghana. Call me Kwame the king." Yet another way to begin the session is to have each person turn to a partner and ask where the partner is from and why the partner wants to learn about HIV. Then each person can tell the group about her new friend.

You can ask people what they have already heard about how HIV is spread and how people get sick from the virus, and about any personal experiences they have had with HIV. This will show what people in the group are most interested in and what they want to learn more about; it gives you a starting place for introducing new ideas. It also helps everyone become comfortable talking in the group. Most important of all, discussing these issues lets the group understand that people have different beliefs and experiences with HIV and AIDS. Some of the people in the group may have HIV. If they feel comfortable talking about their experiences, this can be especially powerful for others. Personal stories make the issues the group will be talking about seem more important to everyone in the group.

Planning a training session: Before you start

Plan goals for your sessions:

>   Design your training to meet the needs of the community.

>   Design the training with the strengths and weaknesses of the group in mind.

>   Choose how many people you want to train.

>   Think about which exercises will work best for the group.

>   Make any learning materials you will need, such as drawings or puppets.

Work with the community to:

>   Choose the place for your session.

>   Choose the best time (time of day, day of the week, and time of year).

>   Make a schedule for the training sessions.

>   Let people know about the meetings.

Once one person begins talking, others usually join in. A feeling of trust and cooperation can be built if everyone feels comfortable speaking. Trust is important. Talking about HIV means talking about sex, drugs, and other sensitive topics. In the beginning, it is easier for the group to answer general questions that do not make people uncomfortable. After talking about sex and HIV in a general way, people will be more comfortable discussing their own experience.

Pay attention to how you state questions. Closed-ended questions are usually not the best way to get a discussion started. For example, asking the group "Does everyone here use condoms regularly?" invites a "yes" or "no" answer and makes those who do not use condoms feel guilty about saying so.

During the course

At the beginning of each class, explain your plan for the day.

Ask the group to make up some rules for the session. Here are some examples:

No one should be pressured to talk about feelings or ideas they are uncomfortable sharing.

Respect everyone's opinions about sexuality. Acknowledge and accept differences of opinion and experience.

Clarify the difference between "I believe" and "It is true that."

Establish confidentiality. Emphasize that no one should talk about other people's personal feelings or experiences outside the group.

Evaluate how your training is going:

Ask people if they are learning what they want to learn.

If they are not, ask for suggestions about how to change the training session to make it better. Should different issues be talked about? Should the training be given in a different way?

After the course

Discuss ways that people can learn more on their own.

Make time for discussion of the course:

Ask the people in the group what they thought about the session and about ways to improve it; talk about successes and problems.

Have group members help organize the next session.

Instead, you might ask, "Why do condoms work against HIV?" Open-ended questions like this invite people to talk and share their ideas.

Notice who is talking in the group. Shy people do not talk very much. In some communities older people hold most of the authority, so younger people may not want to say what they think. In other cultures, the opposite is true. Both younger and older people's ideas are important for learning about HIV.

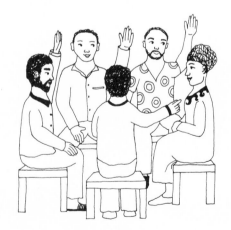

Encourage everyone in the group to speak.

In many communities women will speak less often when they are in groups with men than when they are in groups of women. This is a problem because women's opinions are important when talking about AIDS, and men and women need to talk about HIV together. One of the most important tasks in running a training session is to help everyone share their ideas. Ask each person in the group a question at some time during the training. Do not be afraid of silences. Allow at least three seconds for someone to answer a question—it may seem awkward at first, but more people will express their ideas if they think you are waiting to hear from them. You can ask quiet people to sometimes run the discussion. The idea is to try to bring out different points of view.

Fill in the blanks

People are often embarrassed to talk about sex. Even HIV health workers may be shy about the topic. But it is important for anyone talking about HIV to be comfortable discussing sex and body parts. Humor can help people relax during a training session and allow them to talk more comfortably about these topics. One option is to use a story with blanks. First draw pictures of different body parts used during sex, such as a hand, a mouth, a penis, an anus, breasts, and a vagina. Next, ask the group to give you all the words they know to describe each body part. For example, most people know many other ways to say "penis." Also ask the group for words to describe different sexual acts. Then, write on a chalkboard or piece of paper a story with blanks like the one that follows. Ask each person to read one sentence from the story (or you can read them out loud) and at the blank you point to one of the pictures you have drawn on the board. The person then picks a word from the list to fill in the blank. The next person fills in a word for the next blank. We have included an example below; you can change it to fit your community.

María: Hi, José! What's up? You look tired.

José: Hi, María. I was at home with Tina and I was feeling restless. I asked her if she wanted me to touch her _____ [breasts]. She said no but that I could kiss her _____ [mouth].

María: I understand. I was at the movies with Juan and asked him if he wanted to put his _____ [penis] in my _____ [vagina]. He said he wanted _____ [oral sex].

José: You should have told him that he could _____ [masturbate].

María: Life is complicated!

Helping others lead

Many trainers are surprised to find that there is a lot they can learn from the people in their training sessions. Teaching is sometimes the best way to learn. Medical students in the United States have a saying: "See one, do one, teach one." If someone in the group has special knowledge or skills, she can help teach the group. For example, you can ask a midwife to teach the group about how a baby is born and ways that midwives can protect themselves and their patients from getting HIV. Having people in the training session teach each other helps everyone—including you—learn.

Good trainers often say there is no such thing as a stupid question. If someone has a question, others in the group often have the same one. Try to answer questions when they are raised, rather than at the end of the training session. This way questions are not forgotten along the way and anything that is confusing can be made clear before you move on to the next topic.

Using language and methods that work

Try to teach at a level that is understandable for most of the people in the group. Asking questions will help you know if people understand what you are saying.

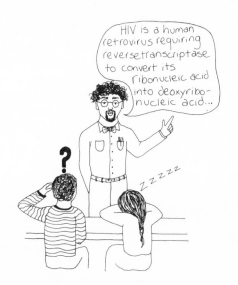

You can change your teaching style to fit the group. Some people learn better from a story or pictures. Others learn better if an idea is written down. Think ahead before trying a new method. For example, if people are not used to seeing drawings that represent a larger-than-life view of an object, you may get unexpected reactions. Drawing a virus on the chalkboard may lead people to believe that viruses are huge. Because they have never seen something that looks like your picture, they may even think HIV does not exist in their area.

Explain words or ideas that are new to the group. Add enough new information each day to keep people interested, but not so much that people are overwhelmed. When possible, give new information in a meaningful way by using practical examples from real life.

Brainstorming

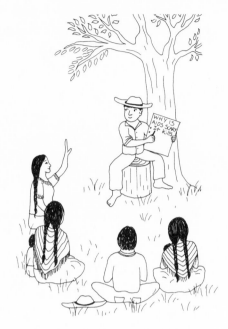

"Brainstorming" is when a group of people get together and share their ideas about how to solve a problem. A brainstorming session about AIDS might start with the question "Why are people afraid of people with AIDS?" The group can talk about people's fears of death and catching the virus. You can talk about these fears and about how HIV really is and is not spread. When brainstorming, write the answers down so that people can see them. Talk about which ideas are most helpful and follow through with the ones that seem best. At the end, discuss the answers and give out tasks for the next meeting. You can use brainstorming to define a problem and to develop a solution.

Using pictures

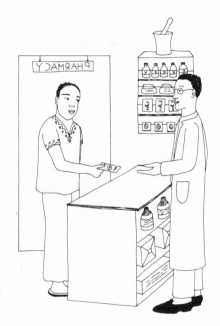

Many trainers use pictures as a means to start a discussion in a group. Pictures are especially useful with people who cannot read, but they can help everyone. Asking the group what a picture means to them will raise different points of view. Let each person tell everyone else what he sees. You should avoid explaining the picture before hearing everyone's ideas; let each person think for himself. For example, you can ask people what they think of a picture of a man in a pharmacy. To get the discussion started, ask a simple question such as, "What is this man buying?" Someone might answer that he is buying condoms, and this might start a discussion about how condoms help prevent the spread of HIV. Someone else might answer that the man is buying medicine, and this might start a discussion about whether there is a cure for AIDS and whether there are medicines for people with HIV and AIDS.

Using role plays

Learning by playing games or watching a play can work better than listening to a lecture. In a role play, people take the role of a character in a difficult situation and act out real-life problems. This helps the people acting and the people watching deal with their own problems. Role plays help people prepare and practice what they would say or do at a difficult time; they bring situations to life. Many situations do not seem complicated when you hear about them, but acting them out while the group is watching can bring out difficulties that appear in real life. Role plays help people to think of creative solutions to those difficulties. Role plays can help people overcome shyness, embarrassment, or fear. You can use a role play to help a person practice telling his partner his HIV test results or asking a partner to have safer sex. Role plays can show the worst and the best things that could happen in a given situation.

A role play

Ask two people in your group to act out a role play involving a husband and wife. One person plays the role of the man, who works five days a week in another town. The other plays the woman, who works in the market at home. The man has started to have sex with another woman from the town where he works. He loves his wife and his girlfriend. Unfortunately, he has recently found out he has HIV. He thinks he got it from his girlfriend. Now he wants to use condoms when he has sex with his wife, but he is afraid that if he tells her about his girlfriend or that he has HIV, his wife and family will disown him. In the role play, the two people can act out the conversations that the man might have with his wife or girlfriend.

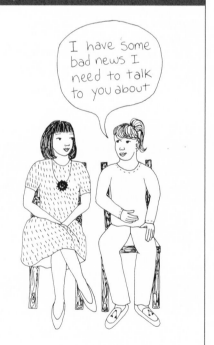

Finally, role plays can help people understand other people's points of view. People in a role play can act their parts for a few minutes and then trade roles. This helps them understand both sides of a problem. It also will help them see how another person would talk about the same problem. Afterward, the group watching the role play can brainstorm with suggestions from their own experience or ideas on how to make talking to each other easier. Two new people from the group can repeat the role play and the group can give more ideas about what they thought worked and did not work.

Serving as an example

Others will learn from your example as a group leader. A leader encourages everyone in the group to participate in learning and teaching. You will set a good example if you show that you are willing to accept your own mistakes and lack of knowledge. When you are genuinely concerned about people with HIV, the people in your training sessions will be too.

Practice what you teach. If you want people to participate, do not spend the entire training session lecturing. Teach through stories, skits, games, and role plays. Think about taking the group to visit an HIV project in another town. Some trainers like to have different activities on different days. For example, Tuesday could be a day for trips to other places to learn from people doing similar work; Wednesday could be a day for working on a play; Thursday could be a day for more traditional lecture-style learning. If the group meets once a week, each meeting might be structured differently. After trying different ways to organize the sessions, you can choose the ways that work best for each particular group. You will know your training is successful when group members are able to teach other people what they have learned.

After the session

Plan for follow-up and support after the training session. Decide how much supervision the new workers will need. How will they start using their new skills? Will they learn best if in the beginning they work with other, more experienced health workers who could give them advice on how they could be better? Will after-work meetings help them learn from common mistakes and experiences? There is always more to be learned. A program of ongoing training will help people continue to learn.

An example of a one-day training workshop for HIV health workers

1. Introductions: Divide the group into pairs. Have the two people in each pair talk to each other about themselves and what they want from the training. Gather everyone in a circle and ask each person to introduce her partner to the group. (15 minutes)

2. Objectives: Discuss what people in the group want to learn by the end of the training. What would they like to be able to do with this information? (15 minutes)

3. Exercise 1: Brainstorm with the group on the ways people can and cannot get HIV. Ask the group members for questions or worries about HIV. The goal is to review how HIV is spread and to help people share their concerns. This exercise helps people talk to each other and make learning goals for the training session. (45 minutes)

4. Presentation 1: Give a presentation about how to identify and counsel patients at high risk for HIV. Include basic information on the spread of HIV, HIV testing, and counseling. (1 hour)

5. Exercise 2: Split into two groups for role plays. Each group can plan a role play, act it out, and then lead a discussion with the whole group. The first play can describe a man and a health worker talking. The man wants an HIV test because he had sex with a woman he visited while traveling (see Chapter 8). The second play can be about a married woman who is worried about being pregnant and having HIV (see Chapter 9). (1 hour)

6. Lunch (1 hour)

7. Presentation 2: Give a presentation about social issues in HIV counseling, including ethnicity, religion, sexual orientation, and drug use. The goal is to help people better understand those from different backgrounds, and to use this information to improve HIV counseling. (30 minutes)

8. Exercise 3: List words used to describe different groups of people in your area. Some of these words will carry negative associations. Talk about the list. The goal is to learn about negative ideas people may have about certain groups of people, and how these ideas can get in the way of HIV education. (1 hour)

9. Exercise 4: Act out another role play to develop different ways to talk about sex. Divide the group into pairs: One person plays a young woman who wants to talk about "safer sex" with a new boyfriend, the second person plays the boyfriend, who would like to have sex with the young woman. The group can watch the two actors and then talk about their behavior. (1 hour)

10. Summary and evaluation: Talk about the training session and about local support for HIV activities. Discuss follow-up training. Have a final round of questions and comments. (30 minutes)

11. Future plans: Ask people in the group to discuss what they plan to do about HIV in their communities. (30 minutes)

Answering Phan's questions

"How do I stir up interest within the group? How do I involve everyone, even the people who usually get bored? What if people are too shy to talk about issues like sex and drug use?"

To stir up interest, it is important that Phan helps the group teach itself about HIV. This means that everyone should have a chance to talk. Phan can ask the group members to sit in a circle and introduce themselves. He can use a picture or a specific question about HIV to get people talking. Different people from the group can write people's questions on a chalkboard. Early in the training, Phan can ask why each person is interested in HIV and AIDS and what he wants to learn. Some people do not like to talk about sensitive issues like sex; in order to make the discussion easier, Phan can have everyone act in role plays. He can break up the large group into smaller groups to talk about different ideas. The small groups can then return to the bigger group and explain what they learned. After the training session, Phan can ask the group what worked, what did not work, and how to make the training better next time.

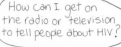

12

Starting community-based HIV projects

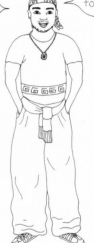

Can you help me teach the students about HIV and drugs?

How can I get on the radio or television to tell people about HIV?

How can I reach teenagers who do not go to school?

Carlos's story

Carlos is eighteen years old. He left his high school in Houston, a city in Texas in the United States. Carlos often got into trouble at school. He used drugs and rarely went to class. His parents finally made him leave their house and Carlos moved into a friend's home. His friend had recently stopped using drugs and he encouraged Carlos to go to a drug treatment program for help. Carlos went to the program and stopped using drugs. Later he attended classes at night and finished high school.

Carlos went to get an HIV test because he was worried that he might have been infected when he shared needles two years before. A week later he learned that he had HIV. He went back to his friends from the drug treatment program and they helped him cope with the bad news. After a while, Carlos decided that he wanted to help teach other young people about HIV so that they would not get the virus like he did. He comes to you for advice: "Can you help me teach the students at my old high school about HIV and drugs? How can I reach teenagers who do not go to school? How can I get on the radio or television to tell people about HIV?"

People working together to address HIV

Many types of organizations are working to stop the spread of HIV and to care for people, families, and communities affected by HIV. Sometimes the government supports these programs. Other times community groups start prevention projects and organize their own efforts to care for those who are infected with HIV or to support families who are affected. Often the government and community groups work together.

To stop the spread of HIV and to provide care and treatment for everyone who needs it, people must take action now and in whatever ways they can. HIV isn't waiting for you to get ready. A community cannot wait for help from a government department, nor can a national government wait for help from the international community.

The rest of this chapter uses prevention programs as examples, but many of the strategies discussed work for care and treatment programs as well.

Here are some questions you can ask that will help you decide whether your area needs a prevention project and what kind of project it should be. You can probably think of other questions that fit your community even better.

- Do people in the community discriminate against people with HIV or AIDS?
- Are there children with HIV in your community? Have their parents died?
- Are there places in your community where HIV is likely to be spread, such as bars, brothels, and clubs?
- Do men or women in your community have more than one spouse or sexual partner at the same time?
- Does your community have condoms? Can people afford to buy them? Are they easy to get? Are people using them?
- If your community has newspapers, radio, or television stations, are they telling people about HIV? If so, are the messages accurate?
- Are schoolchildren being taught about HIV?
- Is blood being screened for HIV?
- Do health care workers understand how to avoid HIV at work?
- Do people know how drugs can spread HIV?
- Are people asking whether AIDS is spread by insects?
- Do people who do tattooing, scarification, acupuncture, and circumcision know how to avoid spreading HIV?
- Do people understand that HIV can be passed from mothers to their babies?
- Are counseling programs available for people who have questions about HIV ?
- Are clinics, hospitals, and healers able to care for people with AIDS?

Community outreach

Community outreach is a way of "reaching out" and teaching the people in a community about HIV and AIDS. Usually this is done in places where people live and work, by people who are members of the community. These people are called outreach workers. They talk with people about what they really want to know about HIV. Outreach workers can inspire and work with a community to start its own HIV project. They are often role models for other people interested in teaching about HIV.

Often, the best counselors are from the community. Their experiences and backgrounds are similar to those of other community members. People know and trust them. It can be a source of pride for a community to have its members actively help others and increase everyone's knowledge. Also, the more a community does for itself and the less it has to depend on outside help, the healthier and stronger the community will become.

There are many examples of successful community-based AIDS projects. Through outreach work, sex workers and former drug users have acted as role models in their communities. Gay communities in many cities of the world have organized strong networks to teach people about HIV.

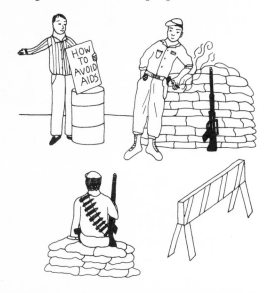

Which projects work?

Thriving community health programs often have these features in common:

They begin small and grow slowly, as the needs and resources of the community grow and change.

They involve the community in each part of the work, from planning to evaluation.

They ask people from the community to take part in the work.

They use leaders whose main interest is serving the community, not advancing their careers or making money.

The people running the programs remain open to new ideas and adapt to the changing needs of those served by the project.

The people involved do not think about health just in terms of the prevention and treatment of disease; they think of each person's social, emotional, and physical situation.

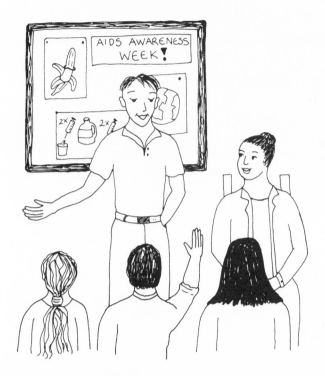

One of the most effective ways to teach about HIV is to have someone who has HIV speak about her experiences to a group of people. When a person with HIV speaks directly to others, she can have a tremendous emotional impact. When she talks about how people can protect themselves from HIV, they will remember what she says. At the same time, she can show that a person with HIV, like anyone else, deserves respect. If the speaker is not a health worker, it may be helpful to have a health worker available to answer difficult questions or to help spark a discussion.

Places to talk to people about HIV

Many people are not comfortable in a clinic or hospital and will not come there to learn about HIV. You can use a clinic for teaching some people about HIV, but be sure to offer other places. This is especially important for people who cannot get to a clinic because of problems with transportation, time, or cost. No single place can be reached by everyone. It is important to bring HIV education to the people, not to make them come to you.

Good HIV outreach programs focus on places where people work, live, and play. Outreach workers have used barbershops, community centers, popular street corners, parks, schools, bars, and brothels. If you know the community, you can have a conversation about HIV with almost anyone almost anywhere. While talking with somone you can share pamphlets, condoms, and bleach kits.

East Palo Alto AIDS Project

East Palo Alto is a small city in California in the United States. It is a poor community surrounded by rich cities. Many families live in East Palo Alto but there are few schools for the children. Many people cannot find work. A number of people use drugs and more and more people are getting HIV.

Some years ago, a few people in East Palo Alto decided that they wanted to stop the spread of HIV. They did not have much money but they had a lot of pride. They decided to teach drug users about how HIV was spread and how they could protect themselves. They knew that they needed to bring the message to where people were: on the streets. The best person to do this was a man named Martin. Martin had used drugs but then stopped; at the time the project started, he had not used drugs for over a year. He felt strong enough to be around people using drugs and not start using them again himself. Martin was known in the community and had many friends. He had a strong desire to help his community and he knew the ways of the streets. Most important, he knew how to talk with people on the streets about HIV.

Martin set up an office in a trailer parked near a place where people used drugs. He got pamphlets about HIV from the state government, had condoms donated by a local clinic, and made "bleach kits" for cleaning needles. On each of the pocket-sized bottles filled with bleach, he and his partner Atieno pasted instructions on how to clean needles and a telephone number people could call for more information on HIV. They explained the project to the police in advance so that the police would not think they were selling drugs.

Martin put the materials in a backpack and went out onto the streets. He started talking to people about HIV and how it is spread. He gave bleach kits to anyone who would take one. Soon he became known as "the bleach man" and people would look for him on the street and call out his name. Before long most of the drug users in the community knew about cleaning needles and about using condoms during sex. Men and women who traded sex for money also learned from Martin. Soon Martin had so much work that he needed help. He went to a local medical school and asked students to help him teach people on the street. They set up a table in a parking lot and passed out condoms, pamphlets, and bleach kits to people passing by. They also tried to give out cookies and bananas so that people would feel comfortable coming by the table—sometimes it is easier to ask for a free cookie than it is to ask for information on HIV.

Martin and the students set up a regular schedule and people began to rely on them for AIDS information and supplies of condoms and bleach. Atieno answered phones at the office and coordinated the project. She talked with church leaders and got donations of supplies. With the help of a local clinic, Martin and Atieno set up a pre- and post-test counseling service for people who wanted to be tested for HIV. The project grew and Martin and Atieno were able to get small salaries from the government for their work. They found it was surprisingly easy to get support for the project once they proved it worked.

Make sure that you choose a place where you feel safe; it will be difficult for you to talk to people if you are afraid. You may not feel comfortable talking about HIV on the street at night in a dangerous part of town, even if this is where you might find the people most in need of information. On the other hand, you may feel safe near a police station, but it probably is not the best place to talk about HIV with sex workers or drug users.

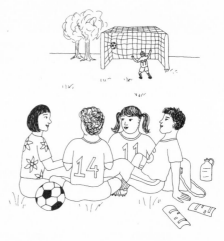

Churches, mosques, schools, hospitals, and organizations like unions or professional associations often have regular meetings of their members. You can ask to give a talk during one of their meetings. You can even talk with sports teams about HIV prevention. Speaking at schools with children and young adults before they are at risk for HIV is especially important. You can work with all of these organizations to help them become involved in HIV prevention.

Do not forget to talk about HIV with health workers. Often physicians, nurses, midwives, traditional healers, and laboratory technicians do not know enough about AIDS. Discussions about HIV will help clear up misunderstandings. People often look to health workers for information about HIV, so it is especially important that they know the truth and teach it to others.

Working with traditional healers

When most people in the world get sick they visit a "traditional" healer. Although we discuss Western medical treatments in this book because they are what we know most about, traditional healers have much to offer in terms of HIV prevention and care.

You can find out who the traditional healers are in your community and where they work. Involve them in your prevention program. It will help you learn more about what they are doing for people with AIDS and help them learn more about what you are doing to prevent the spread of HIV.

In South Africa, each traditional healer has an average of 2,000 visits a year from people seeking health care. In 1991, people in that country started an HIV prevention program that involved training South African traditional healers in how to prevent the spread of HIV. The healers discussed among themselves how to mix Western ideas with their own traditional ideas. They then trained other traditional healers. Information about preventing HIV and treating people with AIDS spread quickly.

In your community, you will find people with different backgrounds, jobs, and lifestyles. HIV prevention programs will work better if they are tailored to reach different kinds of people. Street children, mothers, truck drivers, sex workers, army personnel, migrant farmworkers, and drug users are all at high risk for HIV; help these people create their own HIV prevention programs. If everyone puts creativity and time into designing an HIV prevention program, it will work.

Outreach to people in bars in Bangkok

People in Bangkok, Thailand, organized an outreach program to get information about AIDS to people at high risk. In Bangkok, people who visit bars and work in them are at risk for getting HIV because many people go to bars to meet people for sex. Waiters, bartenders, doormen, and customers all need to know about HIV.

To get started, HIV health workers visited bars and met with people working there. They talked with them and established feelings of trust and familiarity. Then the outreach workers started bringing AIDS information to the bars.

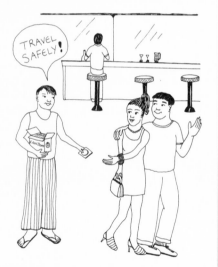

They talked about ways that the bar workers could share AIDS information among themselves and with customers. For example, when a sex worker or customer leaves the bar, a waiter or doorman hands her a condom and says, "Travel safely." The outreach workers also told people where they could get more information outside the bar.

Here are the basic steps used in the Bangkok project:

1. Visit the bars and get to know the people there. Make sure to meet the boss.
2. Learn the rules of behavior at the bar. Always pay your bill.
3. If sex is being exchanged for money, learn how the business works.
4. Learn about the bar workers' private lives: their backgrounds, future plans, relationships, families, sex lives, and health conditions.
5. Learn about the workers' beliefs about HIV and sex.
6. Choose a time and place for HIV education that does not disrupt the day for the workers in the bar.
7. Be flexible; do not push people too hard to change.
8. Show that you do this work because you care about the people working at the bar and want to help them stay healthy.

HIV education in jails and prisons

People who are in jail or prison are at high risk of getting HIV. They often have unsafe sex and share needles when they use drugs. Men and women in jail can be raped either by guards or by other inmates. Prisoners often do not know a lot about HIV because it is hard for them to get good information. In the United Kingdom, former prisoners are trained to talk about HIV. They give talks to people in prison to tell them how to protect themselves from HIV.

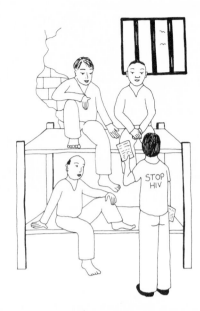

HIV in prison

In Tegucigalpa, Honduras, AIDS is the leading cause of death in the central prison, where in 1998 over 100 prisoners had HIV and 65 had died of AIDS. Officials at this prison are encouraging same-sex marriage among gay inmates to promote monogamy. The officials hope that by being married and having only one sexual partner, men will be less likely to get HIV.

In the United States there are over a million people in prison. The rate of AIDS among prisoners is almost six times that of the rest of the adult population. In spite of this, only 75% of prisons offer AIDS education. This figure is lower than it was a few years ago.

Teaching sex workers about HIV

A sex worker is any man or woman who exchanges sex with multiple partners for money, food, or housing. There are many names for sex workers, such as prostitutes, hookers, and working girls. In some communities sex work is a normal job, while in other places it is illegal and sex workers can be put in prison.

Helping sex workers understand how they can avoid getting HIV is an important part of preventing the spread of HIV. Sex workers should always use condoms to protect themselves and their customers from HIV and other diseases. If a sex worker has a customer who refuses to use condoms, she can suggest a safer practice like oral sex. Sex workers can be great teachers for condom use; some know how to put on a condom without their clients' knowing. Sex workers often have a regular sexual partner (boyfriend, girlfriend, husband, wife) as well as customers. They should be encouraged to have safer sex and to use condoms with that partner as well.

Sex workers can have problems getting health care. They are often victims of discrimination in and outside the health care setting. In some parts of the world sex workers have formed groups to protect their rights. You can help sex workers in your community organize a prevention project. At the same time you can answer questions and encourage discussion about their own HIV risk.

> ### Condoms work
>
> Since 1992, a government program in New Delhi, India has supplied more than 180,000 condoms each month to brothels in New Delhi. In early 1997, the condom supply started to run out. This left nearly 10,000 sex workers at higher risk for getting HIV and other sexually transmitted diseases. People worked hard to get the condoms supplied again.
>
> A few years ago, a group of sex workers in Greece took part in a study. About the same number of sex workers in the study used condoms as did not use condoms. In one year, twelve sex workers who did not use condoms got HIV, while only two workers who did use condoms got HIV. This information was given to sex workers throughout the country. The rate of condom use went up.
>
> In the United States wives and husbands of people who had HIV were asked if they used condoms. These people all got tested for HIV. Eighty-five percent of the partners who did not use condoms had HIV. Only 10% of the partners who did use condoms had HIV. Condoms worked.

Teaching drug users about HIV

Find out whether people in your community inject drugs like heroin and amphetamines (speed). Teach them about how to avoid spreading the virus when they use drugs. Drug users should get their own needles and syringes and never share them. If they cannot do this, they should clean their needles and syringes with bleach before sharing them. Help drug users understand that they should clean needles and syringes that they buy on the street—they may be used and still have HIV in them. (We discuss how to clean needles in Chapter 6.)

People use drugs for many reasons; often these reasons are complex. Some drug users believe that sharing needles builds trust and makes people closer, almost like having sex; they may not want to stop sharing needles. It is difficult to help drug users change their behavior, but it can be done. Some people will change, some will continue to use drugs, but everyone deserves a chance to change. Do not get discouraged.

In most of the United States it is against the law to have needles or syringes that are not prescribed by a doctor. Because of this, drug injectors end up sharing needles. When needles are shared, blood is passed from person to person. This spreads HIV. In San Francisco, California, thousands of people inject illegal drugs. A small group of people interested in stopping the spread of HIV decided to get needles to the people who needed them. They bought clean new syringes and needles and went out on the streets. They traded one new needle for each used one. With the new needles they gave out small bottles of bleach and water to clean the needles between uses. They also talked to drug users about how they could avoid HIV and where they could be tested. The need for clean needles was so great that the workers expanded to five street corners in the city. After a short time they were trading 12,000 syringes a week. A few of the workers were arrested by the police while passing out clean needles. However, the people of San Francisco and doctors and nurses in the city protested in support of the workers. The police commissioner then announced that he would order the police not to bother the workers.

HIV testing as part of prevention

Testing people for HIV can be part of a prevention program. Offering HIV testing can help draw people to your project who might not come otherwise. Pre- and post-test counseling sessions will give you a chance to teach people about HIV. In some communities, local volunteers have been trained as peer counselors and counsel people before and after they get tested for HIV. You can teach people with positive HIV tests how to avoid spreading the virus. You can talk with people with negative HIV tests about how they can stay free of HIV. You can set up regular times when anyone can talk to a counselor about HIV in private. (We talk about HIV counseling in Chapter 8.)

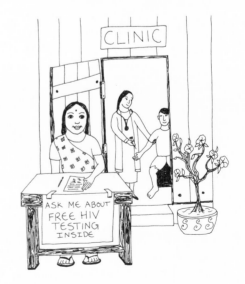

Encouraging people to be voluntarily tested is usually a good idea. It gives people information that can be useful in changing behavior. However, forcing people to be tested can be harmful. Some communities test all people who want to get married, but many people have sex before they get married—testing at the time of marriage is too late! Some countries test all immigrants for HIV, but testing immigrants will not prevent the spread of the virus if the country already has many people with HIV. In fact, it could give people the false idea that HIV is being kept out of the country and that they do not need to exercise safe behavior.

In some places, people have talked about branding or tattooing people who have HIV. Others have suggested that they be quarantined (separated from the rest of society) or put in jail. Carefully think about whether your testing program will be helpful or not. The best testing programs are planned with the help of people in the community who already have HIV and people who are at high risk for infection.

How to create a good message

Deciding that you want to teach people about HIV is only the first step to a prevention program. You also have to think about the *audience* (whom you want to reach), the *message* (what you want to say), and the *medium* (the way that the information is presented). The *audience* could range from street children to health workers. The *message* could range from encouraging people to use condoms when they have sex to telling children not to be afraid of other children who have AIDS. The *medium* could range from fliers to radio announcements, from newspaper articles to songs. The audience, message, and medium all need to be kept in mind. For example, if you want to reach truck drivers, a radio campaign may work well, because people often listen to the radio while driving. The medium matches the audience. If you want to encourage people to get tested for HIV, a poster with complicated medical information about AIDS will not be useful. The people you want to reach

---

Your message about HIV

These are the basic parts of any HIV prevention message. When creating your message, think about them, as well as about whom you want to reach:

Content: what is being said.

Presentation: how the message is laid out, and where (for example, in a poster, in an advertisement, or on the radio).

Tone: the mood of the message (happy, fearful, inspiring, serious, etc.).

Benefits: what a person will gain by learning the information.

---

must understand the message, not be offended by its content or tone, and be attracted to the presentation.

Different people listen to different sources of information. Teenagers may believe facts given by famous rock, movie, or sports stars. Health care workers and professionals trust information from the health department. Parents may be more interested in hearing information from other parents or a trusted health care worker.

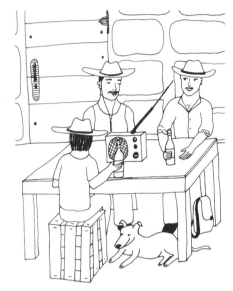

Tone is an important part of any message. Posters in Kenya show a big fist crushing AIDS as a symbol for the power of the community to beat the disease. In one radio advertisement, a mother talks softly to her daughter about the risks of HIV to her daughter's baby. The tone is intimate. It attracts people and makes them listen. Think about who will be hearing the message and tailor it for them. Choose the right medium. Use the right tone.

Focus groups

The best way to create a message that works is to invite people from the community to help you plan your message and choose the best medium. For example, you may want to increase the use of condoms in your community.

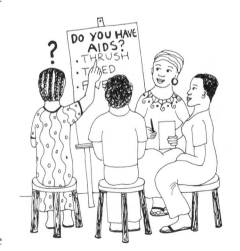

You can meet with a group of people from the community—a "focus group"—and ask them the best way to get information about condoms to people. After several suggestions, the group may decide that posters would be a good medium for spreading the word about condoms. The focus group can help with the words, the picture, and the tone. After you have made the poster, ask another focus group from the community to look at it and give suggestions. Once you know that the

Common misunderstandings about HIV and AIDS

Attitudes about HIV will affect how well your message works. If people do not think that HIV will affect them, then they will not listen to your message. In one part of Tanzania, some people thought that AIDS was caused by witchcraft. They thought that traders in the bordering countries of Zaire, Burundi, and Rwanda used witchcraft to get even with traders who had cheated them. They believed this because at first, most of the people who became ill were traders. People believed that if they were not traders they were safe. Of course this was not true. Traders travel; many got HIV from sexual partners in places where HIV was widespread. Sex, not trading or witchcraft, spread HIV in this part of Africa.

In parts of Africa some people believe that only very thin people have AIDS. In some areas AIDS is called "slim disease." People believe that if they avoid having sex with thin people, they will not get HIV or AIDS. Even though being ill with AIDS can make you "slim," people with HIV can be fat or thin and can give other people the virus no matter how big or small they are.

In one part of Uganda, people thought that if a person had sex just once with someone who had HIV she would get infected. This meant that many people who were married to people with HIV did not get tested and did not practice safer sex because they thought they were already infected. People were encouraged to get tested as part of a study. When the results were shared with the participants, many people who thought they had HIV found out they were not infected. Many of them changed their sexual behavior to lower the chance that they would become infected, or, if they had HIV, to avoid spreading the virus to their partners.

People in the state of Florida in the United States thought that HIV was being spread by mosquitoes, because many people who had HIV lived next to a swamp. People refused to go out at night. They worried that a mosquito bite would give them HIV. Finally, health workers and epidemiologists carried out a study and found out that drug use and sex, not mosquitoes, were spreading HIV. Mosquitoes have never spread HIV.

These examples of misunderstandings about HIV show how important it is to find out what people in your community think about HIV before you begin your prevention program. Then you will know what false information needs to be proven wrong, and who is most likely to need education.

poster is understandable and will work well, you can make copies and distribute them in the community.

Focus groups can help clear up confusing messages. Imagine that you want to design a poster that lists the signs of AIDS. After making a rough draft you show it to a small group of people to see how it works and how it can be improved. Do they understand it? Is it clear? Do they like it, or is it offensive? They tell you that they have never heard of "thrush," one of the signs of AIDS.

You can then change your poster to include a description of thrush as a white, pasty mouth infection. Focus groups help you create a message that is made especially for your community.

How to get the word out

There are many ways to get messages about HIV to people in the community. One way is person to person. By talking with someone you can find out what he already knows about HIV and what you can teach him. Pamphlets, billboards, and radio and television announcements cannot do that. Many people already talk about HIV to each other; they just might not know as much about HIV as someone who has been trained. The more people you talk with about HIV, the more effective their conversations with their friends will be. Each barber, traditional healer, truck driver, taxi driver, and bar worker that you teach about HIV will talk with several other people about the virus. In time the whole community will know something about HIV and AIDS.

Teach community organizations about HIV. Give talks at meetings, show videos, and pass out pamphlets. Members of churches, the police, unions, companies, business groups, the army, and professional groups such as teachers are all interested in HIV and can teach other people about it. Government organizations such as the ministries of health, defense, and finance are other organizations that can teach their members about HIV.

A sample project: Teaching pregnant women about the spread of HIV

Define your target group: Women of childbearing age at a local clinic.

Define your goals: By the end of the training session, women in the group will know that HIV can be spread from mother to baby during pregnancy, birth, and breast-feeding.

Design your materials: Develop a ten-minute training session for mothers waiting at the clinic. Make some visual aids, such as posters, to help explain some of the ideas. Discuss the ways HIV can be spread to babies and what mothers can do to prevent it from being spread.

Evaluate your project: After the session, ask women in the clinic questions about how HIV is spread. This will tell you what they did or did not learn and how you might improve your training.

Talking to people about HIV at work is a great way to reach people. This is especially true if they are given a special break from their work for your talk. On-the-job discussions of HIV can help stop rumors and fears that spread in the workplace. In one small city, people at a telephone company refused to go to work because another worker had HIV. The man with HIV was then fired from his job. One of the workers knew HIV was unlikely to spread on the job and started to teach other workers that they could not get HIV by working with someone who has the virus. The workers went back to work and the man with HIV got his job back.

Creative ways to publicize your message

Over the years people have used hundreds of creative ways to teach about HIV. They have written messages about HIV on car bumper stickers, shopping bags, and T-shirts. They have mailed letters to every household in a city. They have organized puppet shows, community theater, AIDS days, and fairs to bring attention to HIV. At these events musicians, actors, puppeteers, and people from AIDS projects teach the community about HIV. You can use resources from your own community to be just as creative.

Community theater and puppet shows

Community theater is used all over the world to present political issues, educate communities, and provide entertainment. Theater attracts a crowd. It is a break from everyday activities. Community members can write their own play and take part as actors, directors, and stage helpers. They can include a point in the play where people from the crowd can join in. The people in the play can have fun and even laugh at their own mistakes. After the play, people in the crowd may talk about the characters they saw and think about their own lives.

Theater can be used to talk about HIV and private issues such as sex, illness, and drug use. Stories about HIV touch deep emotions, but they can also be funny. A common story is a play about a husband and wife who both have lovers. Neither knows about the other's; they only talk about their lovers with their friends. Many stories can be adapted to different age groups, languages, or cultures. If you put on a play, learn which words are used in the community. For example, in some Spanish-speaking countries, using *la colita*, which mean "private parts," may be better than using the exact words

In the countryside of Thailand, community theater, or maw lum, is used to teach about HIV and AIDS. Maw lum mixes music, dance, drama, and mime. Colorful costumes worn by the actors bring many people to see the play. Since many people in the countryside do not speak Thai, they are not able to understand AIDS messages on television and radio. Maw lum uses the local language instead of Thai. The whole community comes out to watch the play, which is followed by school programs, counseling, and condom distribution.

A common maw lum story is about two young men who leave their village to go to Bangkok to find work. In Bangkok, they visit a brothel. Most of the sex workers have learned to use condoms, but one of the men does not like using condoms. Years later he comes home to the village and starts to have early signs of HIV disease. After time passes he dies of AIDS. The play shows the feelings of his family and friends. The man's wife gets HIV and his children talk about how they feel about their parents' illnesses. They must face the fact that their mother and father are dying and they will have to live with their grandparents. The play also shows the life of sex workers in Bangkok and shows how the sex workers, the brothel manager, and clients in the brothel try to teach everyone to use condoms each time they have sex.

for "vagina" and "penis." In some parts of Zimbabwe, it is less offensive to use *kutsi*, meaning "down there," than to use more specific words.

Puppet shows can also be used to tell a story about HIV. Puppets can be used to speak openly about sex. Small puppets can be beautiful and yet easy to make, and tall puppets that are meters high can attract a large crowd.

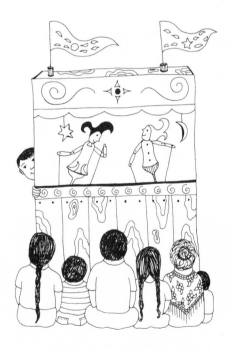

Hotlines

Some communities where many people have telephones have set up a telephone number that people can call to get information about HIV. This is called a "hotline." Hotlines help people get information when they need it, often 24 hours a day. The people who answer the phone need to be knowledgeable about HIV; they also need to know where a caller can get tested for

HIV, receive medical care, or get help when having thoughts about suicide. Educational materials from your project can have your group's hotline number printed on them so that people can call if they need help.

Using the media

There are many ways to use the media to present your message about HIV. The possibilities include print media, like newspapers and magazines, and broadcast media, like television and radio.

"Prudence" condoms in the Congo

In the Democratic Republic of the Congo condoms are now distributed in an attractive package. They are called "Prudence" condoms. Prudence means being careful. The name helps people understand why using a condom is a good idea. Also, the condom package shows a leaping leopard, which is the mascot of the national soccer team. The condoms are sold for a small amount of money in pharmacies, small shops, and on the street.

It was not always like this. In Kinshasa, in 1986, pharmacies only sold condoms in small numbers. They were expensive and rarely used. One study that asked married couples what they used for contraception found out that only 1 of 100 couples (1%) used condoms. In 1987, 200,000 condoms were given away for free and 20% of the men who were asked said they would use them to avoid AIDS. Thousands more condoms were then brought into the country and sold to businesses for resale. Radio advertisements, T-shirts, keychains, printed plastic bags, leaflets, a comic book, and a song were all made about Prudence condoms. After that, almost all of the pharmacies in Kinshasa sold condoms, and they sold 40 times more than they had before. People borrowed ideas that had been used for marketing products in business and used them for social causes. This "social marketing" campaign increased condom use.

Think about the most important parts of your HIV message. Talk about them. Next decide on the best way to get the message out to the community: Radio announcements? Advertisements in the newspaper? Community theater? Pamphlets in medical clinics? Talks at schools? Could someone help you make the posters? Would the radio station give you free airtime? Do you know anyone who works at the local newspaper and would be interested in writing an article about your program? Knowing what medium you are going to use will influence your message and vice versa.

Print media: newspapers and magazines

Newspaper or magazine stories about people with HIV can teach other people about the virus without their even knowing that they are learning. These stories help readers understand the life of a person with HIV. They can make readers sympathetic toward someone with HIV—someone they might have avoided before they read the story. Newspaper and magazine stories also let people with HIV know that they are not alone.

Newspapers in Uganda

In Uganda, some newspapers have regular columns on HIV and AIDS. The New Vision newspaper has an insert called "Saving Youth from AIDS." The insert has stories and information about HIV and can be given out separately from the newspaper.

Another newspaper, called Straight Talk, focuses on changing the way teenagers think about AIDS. The paper was started in 1993 and reaches about one million readers in six languages. Straight Talk openly discusses sex and HIV. It includes articles on sex before marriage and advice columns on AIDS. It tells the truth about sexual myths. The paper encourages teenagers to not have sex at a young age. It teaches sexually active teenagers the importance of condom use.

A newspaper not only provides a way to teach about HIV, but can also give you a chance to find out what people already know. In Kenya, a group made up a list of questions to find out what people in the area knew about HIV. The group then got the questions published for free in the local newspaper. People mailed back their answers, and the group used the information to design educational campaigns.

More people will return a survey or questionnaire if you mention that a drawing will occur in which one of the people answering can win money or a prize (like a bicycle). You can try to get these items donated. Include your program's phone number or address in the newspaper so people can get more information about HIV and your project.

Films and videos

Films and videos are powerful ways of telling a story about someone with HIV. Having a friend who is sick with AIDS is a moving experience. Films and videos can bring this same feeling to people who may not know someone with HIV.

Films and videos are especially useful when limited help is available and when there are language differences. What if only one person at your project

The following is a copy of a survey used to ask people what they knew about AIDS. It might be useful in areas where people do not know a lot about HIV. You can change the questions or add new ones to fit your community.

Please circle the answers you think are right and return the questionnaire to [your group's address].

1. What causes AIDS?
   a. a bug
   b. a bacteria
   c. a plant
   d. a virus

2. How do people get AIDS?
   a. from sharing clothes
   b. from toilet seats
   c. from mosquitoes
   d. from sex

3. Can you tell if someone has AIDS by looking at them?
   a. yes
   b. no

4. Is there a cure for AIDS?
   a. yes
   b. no

5. Will most people with AIDS die from the disease?
   a. yes
   b. no

6. What is one way to avoid HIV?
   a. use condoms during sex
   b. wipe off toilet seats before use
   c. avoid mosquitoes

If you have any questions about HIV, call or visit your local health clinic.

speaks Hausa, but several people who speak only Hausa are interested in being tested for HIV? First, show a video in Hausa on HIV testing. Then the staff member who speaks Hausa only needs to spend time answering questions after the video.

Videocassette recorders (VCRs) are spreading throughout the world and video parlors are quickly becoming popular. Be creative about where you show your videos. VCRs can be used to show videos in the waiting rooms of

Film, video, and television

Film, video, and television work because they are:

Attractive: People like visual images and remember them.

Influential: They are seen by many people and can influence public opinion.

Educational and entertaining: They can combine a message with a story.

Emotional: While telling a story, they can touch people's emotions and change their viewpoints.

Inspiring: They can show role models teaching about HIV.

Cost-effective: They can reach a lot of people at once; they can be copied and used many times.

Portable: VCRs can be used almost anywhere there is electricity.

Some of the limitations of film, video, and television:

Cost: It can cost a lot of money to make a video or buy time on television.

Difficulty: Experience is needed to make a good video or film.

Limited audience: You will not reach people who do not have access to televisions or VCRs.

One-way flow of information: These media do not allow conversation or disagreement.

Mass media work if:

The message is made for a specific target audience, such as teenagers or pregnant women.

The information comes from a source that people like, understand, and believe (such as doctors, basketball players, or musicians).

The presentation gives a clear message that matters to the viewer.

The message tells people how to take action to avoid getting HIV.

The program connects people with other programs that are available in the community.

clinics, in mobile vans, barbershops, schools, and video parlors. If you make a video, make copies and lend them out.

Broadcast media: Television and radio

Television and radio, like film, can bring HIV messages to life. They also reach large numbers of people; that is why they, along with newspapers and magazines, are called "mass media." Millions of people have a television or

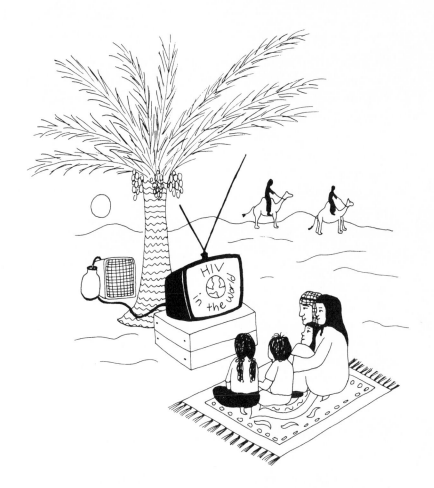

radio in their home. Radios outnumber televisions in most countries, but the number of televisions is growing fast. There are around 1 billion television sets in the world—and 5.5 billion people. Many countries have only one channel. This means that if you show a program about HIV, it will not be missed!

Radio campaigns in Cameroon

National AIDS programs have set up competitions for musicians to make songs about HIV. If the song is catchy and the singer popular, then the radio stations will play it. Often stations will play the song for free, as a public service. In Cameroon, stations played a song called "Le SIDA ne pardonne pas," which, translated, means "AIDS is unforgiving" but also means "AIDS is a fatal disease." It has a catchy tune and people hummed it in the streets. It got people thinking about AIDS. The next step was to teach people how to avoid the virus.

Mass media campaigns are often successful when they use famous people to give a message about HIV or AIDS. People talk about these advertisements. Imagine a poster presenting a picture of a famous cricket player in India: "There were 2.5 million people living with HIV in India in 1997. You can help stop the epidemic and avoid getting HIV by suiting up for the game every time."

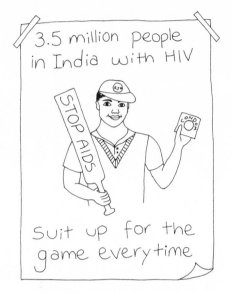

This poster works for three reasons. First, it presents facts about HIV that get the message across: that there are many people with HIV in India, and therefore the person reading the poster should care about his own risk. Second, it shows a famous athlete caring enough about HIV to be on the poster without embarrassment. The viewer need not be ashamed to find out more about HIV. Third, it uses humor to make the issue less depressing and leaves a lasting impression on the viewer. People might ask their friends, "Did you see that funny poster of the cricket player?"

Did our project work?

Here are some questions you can ask yourself after your project has been going for a while:

1. How many people have heard your message?
2. What groups were you trying to reach, and did they hear the message?
3. Have people begun to change their behavior?
4. What did people think of your project?
5. Were the benefits to the community worth the expense?
6. How can the project be improved?
7. What is the most successful part of the project?
8. What is unsuccessful about your project?
9. What would you do differently if you could start over?
10. Would this work in another city or neighborhood?

Answering Carlos's questions

"Can you help me teach the students at my old high school about HIV? How can I reach teenagers who do not go to school? How can I get on the radio or television to tell people about HIV?"

Carlos should think carefully about whether he wants other people to know he has HIV. If he is willing to tell people, then he could teach high school students even more effectively. Teach Carlos about HIV and AIDS and help him learn how to talk to groups of people. Then call up schools in the Houston area and arrange for Carlos to speak with other students about HIV. Have an HIV health worker help him during the talks.

Carlos is also interested in reaching teenagers who do not go to school. A radio advertisement on a popular station is a good way to start. Help Carlos call the local radio station to see if he can make a public service announcement—using free airtime—about HIV. See if someone from the station will volunteer to help him make his announcement. He may even want to go on television. By using radio and television and by talking in the schools, Carlos can teach many young people about HIV.

13

Getting resources for an HIV project

María's story

María runs a women's boarding house called the House of Butterflies in a large city in Peru. Most of the women living in the house are sex workers. Over the past few years, some of the women have become sick with AIDS. The women who are healthy work together to take care of the sick. There have been several attacks against sex workers in the city due to fear and misunderstanding about AIDS, but Maria says the house will always be open to women in trouble, even if they have HIV. The word has spread that anyone with questions about HIV can get information at the house; it has slowly become a community resource center.

At first the women who lived in the house gave their time freely to help those who were ill and to give out information, but this has become difficult because they still have their other work on the streets. More women have become ill and the house needs full-time workers to help the women with AIDS and to give out information. María needs to recruit volunteers and get donations of supplies. She needs money for educational pamphlets, training materials, beds, and medicines. She hopes to find money for salaries for a few people so that they can work full-time. She also wants to reach women who are out on the streets and unable to come to the boarding house for help. María asks several women living in the house to help her find outside support and funds. They have many questions: "Can we teach people in the bars and on the streets about HIV and AIDS? Can we train volunteers from outside the house? Where can we go to get money? How can we write a proposal to ask for support? How can we keep control of the project if we go to big organizations or the government for money?"

Resources

What are resources? Resources are the people and things needed for a project. Tools, land, money, and people are all resources. Some of the best AIDS prevention projects have grown out of communities where resources are scarce. Often people think that their community has nothing, but this is usually not true. People with few resources are forced to be more creative. Finding the resources that are already in the community is often easier than creating new ones. It is true that communities often have little money and are unable to get public or government support; AIDS may have made the community even

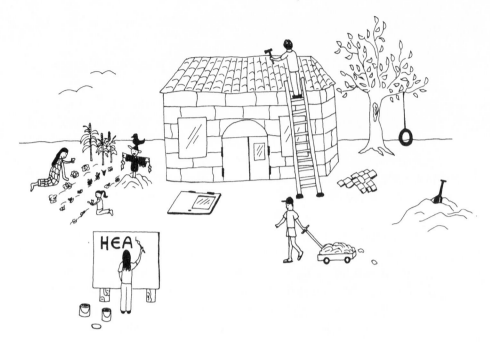

Find resources in your own community first.

poorer. Most health centers have too few staff members, too little medicine, and too few basic materials. With few resources, the job of the health worker becomes more difficult. This chapter will give you some ideas about how to find resources for your community AIDS project. Always look to your community first. You may not realize that it offers some valuable things, such as a place to meet and volunteers with many different skills.

What are the health resources in your community?

People: Healers, health workers, educators, artists, sex workers, parents, and children—anyone with skills who can help with the project.

Skills: People's abilities to teach, heal, plant, harvest, cook, bathe, sing, draw, or write. Some people have the skill to easily learn new skills!

Tools: Hammers, nails, cloth, paper, pens, seeds, shovels, typewriters, and computers—anything that can be used for work.

Land: The ground where a clinic, office, community theater, meeting place, or shelter can be built.

Money: Cash to buy tools, land, or training, or to pay people for their time and work.

Do we need funding?

Many projects could use more money or resources, but often the people involved in the project are too busy with the day-to-day work to look for funding. It takes time to find funding, and it could turn out to be a waste of time to apply for support, especially if the organization you apply to says no to your request. But the time and energy spent can be worth it if you do get support. Think carefully about whether you truly need more resources and have enough time to look for them. Before looking for funding, ask some important questions: Who in the group has time to look for funding? Who in the group knows how to write? Who knows how to prepare a proposal or a request for funding? Who knows how to contact people who work for funding organizations? Which part of the project would most likely be funded?

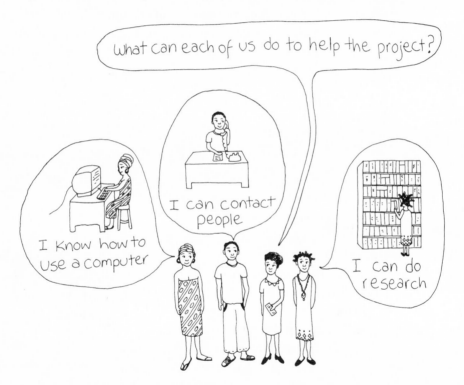

When projects run on the time and energy of volunteers there is often a spirit of closeness. People look after each other. They feel excited by each accomplishment. Getting funding from an outside organization can sometimes change that feeling. Some people may be paid, while others remain volunteers. The people getting your services may demand more when they know that you have money from an outside source. Although there are always needs to be met and the opportunity to expand a project is inviting, funding comes with its own price. It may be helpful to think about this before you plan and write a proposal.

Using local resources first

Support from outside the community often means outside control. That is why it is important to develop local resources before using those of outside organizations. When people from the community control the project, they think of it as their own. Another thing to keep in mind is that if only part of your funds come from outside the community, it will be easier for the project to survive if outside funding runs out.

Keep the resources within your community in mind when designing your project. With experience, your group will learn how to match your project ideas with the resources available in your community. This will make your project easier to run.

Planning the project

Clearly defined projects are easier for an outside organization to support than vague ones. Poorly defined projects are harder to understand and make the people asking for funding seem less organized and trustworthy. When defining your project, be as specific as you can in describing your goals (what your project seeks to accomplish) and methods (how you are going to reach your goals).

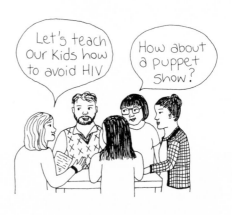

For example, imagine a community where HIV is mostly found among sex workers. People design a project to train two sex workers to teach other sex workers about avoiding HIV. The organizers write a proposal asking for six months of support, including supplies of pamphlets, paper, pens, and condoms, as well as some cash. This is better than asking for US$1000 to "teach people about AIDS." Asking for computers, paper, and assistance to design a questionnaire to ask sex workers about their knowledge about AIDS before and after a year of education is better than asking for "lots of money to fight AIDS in the community." Being vague will leave readers with questions: "How many people in this town have HIV? Who will benefit from the project? How will the group really use the funds? For how long will funds be needed? Does the group have a way of determining whether the situation is improving or getting worse once the project has begun?"

Usually funding is given for a short time. It is easier to find funding for a two-year project than a ten-year project. Showing that the money or supplies were used well and that you are reaching the project goals makes it more likely that you will get more funding when the original money runs out.

Before the money and supplies arrive, the group should talk about how they will be used. This will help prevent future arguments over their use. One way to manage funds is to have a small group of community members oversee how they are used. This project committee should include people with different backgrounds; people with experience in business, health care, community organizing, or religion all make good committee members. People who will be helped by the project should also be on the project committee. Committee members can help find funds for the project, volunteer their time, or donate materials. They should also help with long-term plans for the project.

What does your community need most?

Once you have described or defined your goals, the next step is to decide which parts of the project most need funding. Project members can get together and draw up a list of needs. The list can be numbered with the most important first. You can look at projects in other communities for examples of successes and failures. You may want to talk to other groups about how they decided which needs were most important in their communities.

Next you can think about how you will get the work done. What type of work is involved? Who will need to be trained, and how will they be trained? Will the project include radio advertisements, pamphlets, theater, public speaking, or one-on-one counseling? By deciding on your methods, you will be able to see who could best help you, and who would be most interested in funding you.

María and the women of the House of Butterflies became interested in caring for the sick after seeing so many people with AIDS in their community. They also wanted to stop people from getting HIV. The group talked about their needs and hopes for a project and made this list of goals:

1. Provide care for those who are sick with HIV.
2. Teach the sex workers in the boarding house about HIV and ways to prevent its spread.
3. Teach sex workers on the streets and in bars about HIV.
4. Teach clients of sex workers about HIV and ways to prevent its spread.
5. Teach health care workers not to be afraid of people with HIV.
6. Teach people in the community about the importance of the rights of sex workers and people with HIV.

The group decided to have two projects: First, caring for sick women in the house; second, teaching sex workers and their clients about HIV. To increase their knowledge of the medical aspects of HIV and AIDS, they asked a trainer from Peru's National AIDS Program to help train three sex workers. Next they asked themselves a series of questions: "How can we reach sex workers and clients on the streets? Should we go to the streets and bars most commonly visited by sex workers? What further training would the sex workers need to do outreach? Would they be able to train other women and men to be new outreach workers? Are any clients willing to become outreach workers? Could the local radio station air messages about HIV? Can we find funds for testing and counseling?"

Many of the women already knew a lot about safer sex and avoiding HIV. These women were also well known in the community, which made them the best people to teach others. The outreach program would start by doing a survey to see what fears and knowledge people had about AIDS. The group planned to use educational messages on the radio station played in local bars. The trained outreach workers would talk one-on-one about HIV in the bars and streets. Women from the group also planned to pass out written materials and condoms during hours when they were not working. Later, the group would do another survey to see if people in the community had learned something about HIV.

Making a budget

Make a list of what you will need for your HIV or AIDS project. Include such things as people's time, transportation, supplies, educational materials (such as pamphlets), and radio airtime. Do not forget to include the time that will be spent by volunteers, as well as other donated resources. Make three columns next to your list of items (see the "Budget" figure on p. 179). In the first column—costs—put the cost for each item. In the second column—community contributions—write the amount that your project already has, or will be able to get without outside help. Add up the items in each column to make a total. In the third column—funding requested—subtract the community contributions column from the costs column. This will be the amount you still need for the project, so it will be the total amount of money requested.

Thinking about how much money you will need will help your group decide on which organizations to go to for support. Sometimes, if a project's budget is too big, it can be divided into smaller parts, and requests can be sent to different organizations for partial funding.

Budget
- Supplies $25
- transportation $50
- copies of training manuals $15
- condoms $75
- radio airtime ?
- posters $20
- salaries $

Types of funding organizations

Many types of organizations support health and HIV-related efforts. Sources of funding include governmental organizations, nongovernmental organizations (also called private voluntary organizations), and private individuals. There are national and international organizations. International agencies give larger sums of money but are usually much harder for community-based organizations to reach.

Government agencies are likely to give support to established projects. This makes it difficult for new community organizations to obtain funding from them. Luckily, some countries have a national AIDS organization that will give money to small projects. Nongovernmental agencies will fund small projects; these groups include aid organizations like Médecins du Monde, International Development Exchange, Family Health International, and UNICEF. Finally, private sources, such as wealthy people or corporations, may be willing to donate money or supplies.

Finding sources of funding can be the hardest part of getting support. It is difficult to know if someone might be willing to support your project. Your national AIDS program might be a good source of information about funding

Different types of funding sources
Governmental organizations, such as ministries of health and national AIDS programs
Nongovernmental organizations (NGOs) or private voluntary organizations (PVOs), such as religious organizations, the Red Cross and Red Crescent, and OXFAM
Multinational aid agencies, such as the World Bank, UNICEF, and UNAIDS
Bilateral government organizations, such as the United States Agency for International Development (USAID), the Swedish Internal Development Agency (SIDA), or the Overseas Development Agency (ODA)
Private foundations, such as the Ford Foundation, International Planned Parenthood, or Family Health International
Individuals or corporations willing to donate their own money or resources

organizations. Keep a list of the names and contact people of each organization in order to apply for support when you need it.

Different funding organizations support different kinds of work. Some organizations support only research, others only education. Some support people's salaries, while others support material costs. Some organizations support only established government projects, while others are looking for grassroots community projects. Some organizations have special groups in mind, such as poor communities, women, students, or children. Each organization may support slightly different types of projects, so it is important to think about whom to approach for support. Knowing who will read your proposal and what their special interests are will help you get funding. Learn about the organization by writing or talking to people.

Look to people you know for support. Sometimes mentioning the names of people you have worked with who are familiar to an organization will help you win funding. A well-written proposal helps people understand how the project will work even when you are not there to explain it to them.

What is a proposal?

Now that you have decided on a project, the methods you will use, and the resources that are needed, it is time to begin writing a proposal. A proposal is a paper that describes the project and asks for support. It presents the needs and goals of the project. It also describes a plan of action. A proposal asks for support or funding and promises to carry out the work.

Writing a good proposal

A proposal should be well organized and easy to understand. It should be easy for readers to understand the goals of the project. They should be able to understand how the project will be done and believe that the project can be done. A proposal should answer most of the questions that readers will have.

The first few drafts of a proposal are often written by hand, with a pencil, to allow for changes. Correct spelling errors by using a dictionary and having friends read the rough draft. Leave space in the margins for comments or notes. The final version should be typed (with a typewriter or computer) on white paper. How a proposal looks makes a difference as to whether it will be funded. The final version should be well organized, clearly printed, and without spelling or grammatical mistakes. This will keep the readers' attention on the content of the proposal and not on the errors.

Parts of a proposal

In this section we will describe the parts of a proposal. The boxes along with the text will show examples from the House of Butterflies. Your proposal may be different, but most people choose to include some or all of the following basic parts:

Cover letter

Title page

Table of contents

Summary (optional)

Introduction and background

Objectives

Methods

Evaluation

Conclusions

Appendix

Timeline

Budget

Personnel responsibilities/qualifications

Bibliography

Curriculum vitae or résumé

Cover letter

A cover letter sets the tone for the proposal. Use a confident tone. The letter introduces what the project is about and why it is needed. It briefly describes

---

Cover letter

April 2, 2000

House of Butterflies
Community AIDS Resource
Center
San Luis, Peru
Tel.: 234519

Women's International Development Exchange*
Regional Office
Lima, Peru

Dear [name of person]:

    I run a community-based HIV resource center for educating sex workers and their clients in San Luis. Juan Pérez suggested that I contact you because of your organization's interest in supporting grassroots organizations that focus on groups of people at risk for HIV infection and with limited access to resources. Sex workers and their clients frequently fall into this category, as they are often poor and do not identify themselves as being at risk for HIV.

    Over the last few years we have successfully converted a boarding house for sex workers into a support network, drop-in center, and informal care facility for women with HIV and those wanting health information. The household has cared for more than fifteen people with AIDS, using healthy boarders as volunteers. We have provided basic counseling for over 100 sex workers needing information about how to protect themselves and their clients and partners from HIV. The House of Butterflies is in a unique position to become a specialized health and educational resource for a wider group of people in San Luis. Enclosed is a proposal describing our specific objectives, methods, and budgeting needs for creating a successful outreach program.

    Please contact me or Catia Oscos for any further information. I would be happy to arrange a visit to our project if you have the time. I will contact you in two weeks regarding our proposal. Thank you for your time and consideration.

Sincerely,

María Ramos
Director

*This is not a real organization; we made it up!

---

the people who will participate in the project. It can tell a funding organization why you chose to give them the proposal. It should show that you understand the work of the funding organization. If you mention a person who recommended the organization, the person who receives it may read your proposal more favorably. Your letter should also mention any previous projects that your group has done. A cover letter should usually be no more than one page. If your group has its own stationery, use it for this page.

Title page

The cover letter is followed by the title page. This gives the project title, the name of your group, the name of the funding organization, and the date.

Title page

A Community-Based AIDS Resource Center
for the Education of Sex Workers and Clients

House of Butterflies Community AIDS Resource Center
San Luis, Peru
Telephone: 234519

Submitted to:
Women's International Development Exchange
Regional Office—Lima, Peru
Central Office—San Francisco, California, USA

April 2, 2000

Table of contents

A table of contents is a guide that helps readers find their way through the proposal. It is a list of headings and subheadings with page numbers. This

Table of contents

House of Butterflies
Community AIDS Resource Center

Table of Contents

helps readers locate specific parts of the proposal. (The table of contents in the front of this book is an example.)

Summary

The summary briefly explains to the reader the background and objectives of the project. It should be short, rarely more than two pages. Sometimes people will not have time to read your entire proposal. The summary gives them the information they need to have a general idea of your proposal.

Introduction and background

The introduction sets the stage for the project. It presents in more detail the background of the project and includes the history of the problem, attempts to fix it, and why further efforts are needed. Proposals often mention past projects involving the same field of work done in similar areas. They may discuss the successes or weaknesses of these projects and how the current project will build on the good points and avoid the mistakes. The introduction establishes the need for the project and how it will serve the community. You can describe the community you will be working with and the people who will participate in the project. You can discuss what other projects were considered by your group and why this one was chosen.

Objectives

In this section, you present the objectives of the project in a brief numbered list. This list states specific goals the project will attempt to accomplish.

Objectives

1. To identify the attitudes, knowledge, and practices of people in our community regarding HIV and AIDS.
2. To train three sex workers and one client to do outreach HIV education appropriate for the community.
3. To distribute 30,000 condoms and 5,000 educational pamphlets on the street and in bars. To meet with at least 300 sex workers and 5,000 clients to talk about HIV and AIDS. To answer their questions about HIV, including how to prevent the spread of the virus and how to get tested.
4. To recruit further interested and knowledgeable community members willing to be trained to work in educational and household HIV/AIDS care efforts.

Methods

The methods section describes in detail how the project will be carried out. Usually, the more detailed a methods section, the better. This convinces a reader that you have planned each step involved in the work.

The methods section should describe how you will include feedback from the community in your project from the begining to the end. If you are planning a survey, you should describe it and how it will be carried out. The methods section must be specific enough to address what type of survey you will perform (for example, written questionnaire, personal interviews, open conversation with observations), the length and type of questions you will ask (a sample questionnaire could be added to the appendix), and how you will train interviewers. If you plan to use a laboratory or clinic, you should describe the tests that will be used. Even if you are not sure of the exact details yet, which is common, describe the most likely situation. No one will fault you for making some necessary changes later.

Evaluation

The evaluation section describes how you will study the results of the project to see if it worked. There can be evaluations of the project at the beginning (for example, to test a questionnaire or pamphlet to see if the language is understandable), in the middle (to see how you are doing), and at the end (to check on the overall effects and success). This section states whether you will present a report of the results to the community or local officials. Funding organizations generally require a final report because it shows them that their money was used well.

Sometimes two different types of evaluation are used, process evaluation and impact evaluation. Process evaluation is a measure of how many of the tasks you set out for your project were accomplished. This might include the number of people trained, the number of sex workers counseled, or the number of condoms distributed. Impact evaluation is a direct measure of the effects you wanted to achieve. This might include a lower percentage of sex workers at the House of Butterflies having STDs than last year, or a lower number of sex workers becoming newly infected with HIV. Impact evaluation is often hard to do well, but it can be very rewarding to see good results.

Conclusions

This section explains how the project will serve the community and summarizes the proposal.

Appendix

This part of the proposal includes supporting explanations that are too lengthy to fit into the written text. You can think of the appendix as a reference section for more information. It may include sample questionnaires, diagrams, sample posters, etc.

Timeline

The timeline divides the work of the project into stages, such as development, education, and assessment. It explains how much time will be needed for each part of the project.

Budget

The budget is a list of expenses for the project. It should list individual items and their cost, as well as a total of all the expenses. If two countries are involved, you should list expenses in only one type of currency. The budget should use realistic estimates. Both the budget and related comments say something about the organization of the project. Most funding organizations

Timeline

Development   1–6 months
1. Create a questionnaire on AIDS-related knowledge, attitudes, and practices in the community.
2. Choose and train community members for interviewing and educator jobs.
3. Practice using the questionnaire in small groups to improve it.
4. Evaluate the best community settings for outreach HIV education.
5. Prepare radio spots featuring musical AIDS prevention messages.
6. Test and revise the questionnaire and educational materials.
7. Interview sex workers and clients in the community using the new questionnaire.

Education   7–18 months
1. Start an outreach educational program on local streets and in bars.
2. Start one-on-one and small-group education and counseling.
3. Distribute educational pamphlets and condoms.
4. Play an AIDS prevention message on local radio stations.
5. Write a play and use a local theater to present AIDS prevention messages to the community.
6. Plan a special fund-raising night at the local theater to raise money for the House of Butterflies AIDS care effort.
7. Recruit new community members to train and work at the House of Butterflies center.

Evaluation   19–24 months
1. Continue the educational program in local streets and bars.
2. Interview sex workers and clients in the community about their knowledge and practices regarding HIV.
3. Evaluate and compare the results of the interviews.
4. Write up results for members of the boarding house and local community.
5. Write a final report to the funding organization.

Total time   24 months

will know if a budget is exaggerated and will only give money for what seems essential. However, it is not wise to ask for too little money, either. You may think that a smaller amount will more likely be funded, but if you ask for too little support, you may not have enough money to carry out the project.

When describing the budget in your proposal, you should mention how the money will be controlled. Often people open a bank account that requires the signature of three people from the project to cash a check. A person can

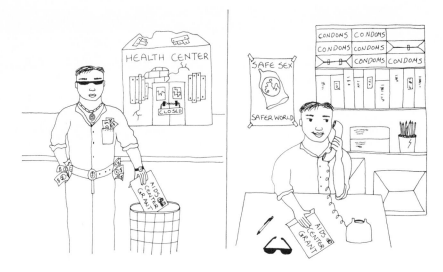

Make sure the money for the project is spent on the project.

take on the task of managing the finances. This will help the funding agency (and you) feel more comfortable that the money is going to the right places.

Personnel responsibilities/qualifications

The personnel responsibilities section includes the job title and the responsibilities that go with each job position in the project, including volunteer positions. For example, you may need a nurse to care for sick women in the House of Butterflies. You could list the job as "Part-time Nurse" and the responsibilities as visiting the house three times a week (four hours each visit), bringing medicines to those who need them and providing basic nursing care for the women.

Bibliography

A bibliography (list of references) is a list of any articles, books, or personal communications that were used to help write the proposal. Usually the authors of the books and articles are listed in alphabetical order, from A to Z (the resources list at the end of this book is an example). This allows readers to obtain further information if they are interested. Many proposals do not have a list of references, but if you include one, it will show that your project was well researched and that you have the information needed to carry out the project.

Budget			
Description	Cost in US$	Community contribution requested	Funding
Materials			
Donated office, 2 rooms	—	—	00
Copying training manual (60 pages x 10 copies)	30	10	20
Copying questionnaire (10 pages x 200 copies)	100	35	65
Office supplies (paper, pens, stapler)	200	70	130
Donated chalkboard (x 2 for training)	—	—	00
Table (1) and chairs (10) (for training)	120	60	60
Pamphlets (5 x 800 copies each)	200	80	120
Condoms (discounted, 4,000)	200	80	120
Poster paper (40)	20	7	13
Radio airtime (partially donated)	100	20	80
Postage and telephone	40	15	25
T-shirts for volunteers (x 40)	200	50	150
Personnel			
Community volunteers (40)	—	—	—
Trainer from regional AIDS program (x 2 wks.)	400	100	300
Full-time salaries 4 outreach workers	20,000	3,000	17,000
Half-time salaries 2 interviewers	2,400	400	2,000
Total	**$24,010**	**$3,927**	**$20,083**

This section of a proposal lists the job qualifications of the people who will be leading the project. This is often done in the form of a curriculum vitae (CV) or résumé, which lists work experience, education, community service, and special skills (language, artistic, or counseling skills). This information shows the funding organization that the people involved in the project are qualified to do the work. CVs are not needed, however. Many projects are led by people who do not have formal training. If that is the case, you may want to write a paragraph describing each person's experience and skills that would benefit the project.

Keeping contacts active

If you are given funding, it is important that you communicate with the organization that is supporting you. It will want progress reports and will usually tell you how often. This will let the funding organization know how the project is going, and it will help you keep track of your efforts.

It is also important to keep the community interested in and supportive of your project. Part of the project should include asking for ideas from the community about how to make the project better. This can be done by working closely with your group of community advisors and contacts.

What happened to María and the House of Butterflies?

"Can we teach people in the bars and on the streets about HIV and AIDS? Can we train volunteers from outside the house? Where can we go to get money? How can we write a proposal to ask for support? How can we keep control of the project if we go to big organizations or the government for money?"

The House of Butterflies finally did get support from the Women's International Development Exchange for its educational project. The women then wrote a new proposal to request money for support services for the people with AIDS living in the boarding house. They submitted this proposal to the Ministry of Health's AIDS Program Office. The ministry gave the group some money. In addition, Maria and the women were able to raise money by performing cabaret theater in local nightclubs. Two wealthy people who saw the shows and heard about the program on the radio gave money for the House of Butterflies project.

Many people from the community came to volunteer at the boarding house. This gave the women a break from their work caring for those with AIDS. Through the project the women living in the house gained new skills in teaching, interviewing, management, and health care. The educational program was a success. People's new knowledge of HIV and AIDS led them to use condoms more often, and fewer sex workers got HIV. Most important, the women gained pride in themselves and their project. The community began to understand the House of Butterflies and the women living there. The acts of violence against them stopped.

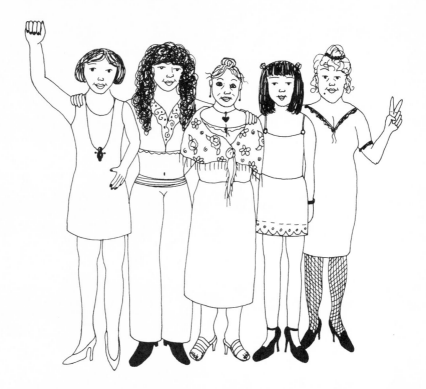

The women faced many challenges after getting the funding. The people being cared for by the project became more demanding. The roles of people in the program changed. In some ways the house felt less like a small community. María, after years of being something like a much-loved mother, landlady, housemate, and friend, said that "people demand things now because they say the ministry of health gives the house money. People want a lot. It is a big change from when we paid for all of it ourselves and everyone was grateful." All in all, though, most of the women in the House of Butterflies continued to feel good about their work.

Appendix

Treating advanced HIV disease: medicines for HIV, and common infections and their treatments

Medicines for HIV

Cotrimoxazole

Antiretroviral therapy (ART, ARV, or HAART)

Opportunistic infections

Skin diseases

Eye diseases

Nerve and brain problems

Mouth problems

Diseases of the gut

Sinus infections

Chest diseases

Blood disorders

Sexually transmitted diseases

HIV and pregnancy

Pain

Vaccines

Medicines for HIV

HIV cannot be cured but it can be treated. Medicines can quickly and dramatically improve the health of a person with HIV. It is common for a person who was very underweight and sick to gain weight, feel stronger, and have many fewer opportunistic infections within a few months of starting

HIV medicines. People who take medicines to treat HIV live for many more years than people who have no access to these drugs. Medicines can also help prevent the spread of HIV from a mother to her baby.

This section explains a few combinations of medicines that can directly treat HIV, as well as how to use cotrimoxazole, which can prevent many opportunistic infections. After this section we discuss opportunistic infections and their specific treatments.

Cotrimoxazole

Taking cotrimoxazole daily can prevent many serious infections and prolong the lives of adults and children with HIV. It prevents malaria, diarrhea, pneumonia, and a brain infection called toxoplasmosis. Fortunately, cotrimoxazole is a common antibiotic available all over the world and rarely causes bad reactions. If a person develops a mild skin rash from cotrimoxazole, she or he can slowly increase the dose of the medicine, which lessens the chance that the reaction will occur again. If a person gets a serious skin reaction, including peeling of the skin or involvement of the mouth, lips, or vagina, then cotrimoxazole should be stopped, the person should seek medical care, and the drug should not be restarted.

For a daily preventive dose, give adults (anyone over 15 years) trimethoprim/sulfamethoxazole 160 mg / 800 mg (2 single strength tablets) once a day. See the chart below for doses for children.

Cotrimoxazole dosage for HIV infected or exposed children				
Age	Dosage	By liquid, 40 mg/200 mg in 5ml syrup	By pediatric tablet 20 mg/100 mg	By single strength adult tablet 80 mg/400 mg
For children age 6 to 14 years old	80 mg trimethoprim/ 400 mg sulfamethoxazole once a day	10 ml	4 tablets	1 tablet
For children 6 months to 5 years old	40 mg trimethoprim/ 200 mg sulfamethoxazole once a day	5 ml	2 tablets	½ tablet
For babies less than 6 months old	20 mg trimethoprim/ 100 mg sulfamethoxazole once a day	2.5 ml	1 tablet	¼ tablet
Babies of HIV-positive mothers should receive cotrimoxizole from birth. If you find later that the baby does not have HIV, you can stop the cotrimoxazole.				

Antiretroviral therapy (ART, ARV, or HAART)

Medicines that directly fight the HIV virus are called antiretrovirals (ARV). HIV is a type of virus called a retrovirus. Antiretrovirals fight retroviruses. For antiretrovirals to work effectively, a number of them should be given in combination. The combined use of these drugs is called antiretroviral therapy (ART), or Highly Active Antiretroviral Therapy (HAART).

In most cases, once a person starts ART, she must continue to take these medicines for the rest of her life. Stopping and starting again can cause resistance to the medicine.

There are a number of challenges that make providing ART difficult:

- The biggest challenge of ART is that most people have no access to it. For many years, companies that made these medicines charged as much for them as they could. Since activists around the world and certain local governments have put strong pressure on these companies to make drugs available to poor people, it is now possible for poor countries to buy drugs at lower prices, or to make generic drugs. Generic drugs are made locally and are much cheaper. As the drugs have become less costly, some international initiatives have begun to provide funding to distribute them. But these efforts are still not enough to provide medicines for everyone who needs them.
- For ART to work well, people must take a combination of drugs and continue taking the drugs for their whole lives. Taking more than one drug at a time can be confusing. If the first combination does not work or causes health problems, the person with HIV may need to switch to another set of drugs.

Before giving ART

ART may not be safe for people with certain health problems. For example, a person with liver disease may not be able to use some of these medicines because they can cause hepatitis. People with HIV should have a physical exam and medical history before starting ART.

HIV medicines are probably safest and most effective if they are given after a person's HIV disease has progressed to a certain stage. If you can test the person's CD4 count, start ART when the person's CD4 count is between 200 and 350 cells/mm^3 (or if the person's CD4 count is less than 200 when you first test the person).

For children 18 months old and older, start ART when the child's CD4 percentage is less than 15%.

If CD4 cell counts are not available, you can use a total lymphocyte count or the stage of the person's disease to decide whether to put the person on ART. The World Health Organization (WHO) has developed a list with symptoms for 4 stages of HIV to help with this decision (see the next page).

ART treatment

There are a number of different combinations of medicines that can treat HIV effectively. This book gives the treatments that are most available and effective at the time this book is being printed (January 2006). No matter what medicines you give, remember that you must give a combination of at least 3 medicines (treating HIV with only one or two medicines is not effective) and some combinations of medicines are available as one pill. This makes medicines easier to take and less expensive. Two combined pills are Combivir, a combination of lamivudine and zidovudine, and Triomune, a combination of lamivudine, stavudine, and nevirapine.

It is important to consider several questions when deciding what combination of medicines to have available in a clinic or to give to an individual.

- What medicines are available and affordable where I live? Are these medicines likely to be available in the coming months and years?
- Is a combination pill available for some or all of these medicines?
- What are the side effects or requirements of the medicines?(For example, some medicines need to be refrigerated; some must be taken with food.)
- Are laboratory tests needed to check if the drug is causing problems for the person taking them?
- Is the person taking rifampicin (a TB medicine) or other medicines that could be dangerous to combine with certain ART medicines?
- Is the person pregnant now or planning to become pregnant? Certain antiretrovirals are not safe in pregnancy.
- If you are giving medicine to a child, how will you give it? Is a liquid available? If not, you may need to open a capsule (though not all capsules may be broken open), or crush a pill (dividing it, if necessary, to get the right dose). You can mix the powder or capsule contents with water or a small amount of food and feed it immediately to the child.

WHO Stages of HIV Infection

Stage 1
- No symptoms.
- Persistent swollen lymph nodes (generalized lymphadenopathy).
- Normal level of activity.

Do not give ART.

Stage 2
- Weight loss of less than 10% of body weight.
- Minor mucocutaneous problems (seborrheic dermatitis, prurigo, fungal nail infections, recurrent oral ulcerations, angular cheilitis).
- Herpes zoster within the last five years.
- Recurrent upper respiratory tract infections (bacterial sinusitis).
- Normal activity level.

Do not give ART unless the total lymphocyte count is below 1200 cells/mm^3. (Total lymphocyte count means a white blood cell count per high-powered field multiplied by the percentage of lymphocytes.)

Stage 3
- Oral candidiasis (thrush).
- Oral hairy leukoplakia.
- Pulmonary TB within the past 12 months.
- Severe bacterial infections (pneumonia, pyomyositis).
- Weight loss greater than 10%
- Diarrhea lasting more than 1 month.
- Fever lasting more than 1 month.
- Bedridden less than half every day during the last month

Give ART to an adult or child in this stage of disease.

Stage 4
- Extra-pulmonary TB.
- Kaposi's sarcoma.
- Cryptococcal meningitis.
- Cerebral toxoplasmosis.
- Cryptosporidiosis with diarrhea for more than 1 month.
- Cytomegalovirus disease of an organ other than liver, spleen or lymph nodes.
- HIV wasting syndrome.
- Pneumocystis jiroveci pneumonia.
- Toxoplasmosis of the brain.
- Herpes simplex virus infection, mucocutaneous for more than 1 month, or visceral for any length of time.
- Progressive multifocal leukoencephalopathy.
- Any disseminated endemic mycosis (histoplasmosis, coccidioidomycosis).
- Candidiasis of the esophagus, trachea, bronchi or lungs.
- Atypical mycobacteriosis that has spread throughout the body.
- Non-typhoid Salmonella septicemia.
- Lymphoma.
- HIV encephalopathy.
- Bedridden for more than half of every day during the last month.

Give ART to an adult or child in this stage of HIV disease.

Here are a few combinations of drugs that work well and are available in many places.

ART for adults

Give this combination 2 times a day, every day:
- stavudine (d4T) 40 mg, and lamivudine (3TC) 150 mg, and nevirapine (NVP) 200mg

This set of drugs is usually available in a combined dose pill.

(If the person weighs less than 60 kilograms, give 30 mg d4T instead of 40mg.)

If the person has numbness or a burning feeling in their arms or legs
(peripheral neuropathy) — or cannot take d4T for some other reason,
give this combination 2 times a day, every day:
- zidovudine (AZT) 300 mg, and lamivudine (3TC) 150 mg, and nevirapine (NVP) 200mg.

If the person has liver problems, TB, is taking rifampicin, or cannot take NVP for some other reason, give this combination 2 times a day, every day:
- stavudine (d4T) 40 mg, and lamivudine (3TC) 150 mg, and efavirenz (EFV) 200mg

(If the person weighs less than 60 kilograms, give 30 mg d4T instead of 40mg.)

Note: nevirapine (NVP) can cause liver problems and rashes. To avoid these problems, give NVP 200 mg only once a day for the first 2 weeks — then increase to 200 mg twice a day.

EFV should not be given to women in the first 3 months of pregnancy, or women who may become pregnant.

Pregnant women and newborn babies

Pregnant women with advanced HIV should take ART to protect their own health. ART is also effective in preventing transmission of HIV to infants.

ART is usually safe for pregnant women, but certain medicines should not be given. For example, EFV can cause birth defects in the child. Women of childbearing age who are using EFV should use birth control. Also, pregnant women should not take d4T and didanosine at the same time because these two drugs can be toxic to the developing fetus when they are combined.

A baby born to a mother with HIV should receive:
- 2 mg oral suspension of nevirapine (NVP)/kg by mouth
  one time within 3 days of the birth
  And
- 4 mg oral solution zidovudine (AZT)/kg by mouth
  2 times a day for the first 7 days of life.

If the mother was not taking ART during pregnancy because she could not get the medicines or because she did not yet need the drugs to treat her HIV, she should take 200 mg nevirapine (NVP) one time at the beginning of labor.

Babies of HIV-positive mothers should also receive cotrimoxazole (see page 184).

ART for children

AIDS should be suspected in an infant or child who has at least two major signs and two minor signs and no other known causes of immunosuppression.

Major signs of AIDS in children

- Weight loss or failure to thrive
- Chronic diarrhea for more than 1 month
- Prolonged fever for more than 1 month

Minor signs of AIDS in children

- Generalized lymphadenopathy (lymph nodes larger than ½ cm in at least two sites)
- Candidal infection in mouth and throat
- Repeated common infections (ear, throat, etc.)
- Persistent cough for more than one month
- Generalized skin infections
- HIV infection in the mother

Children under 18 months old: A sick child who is diagnosed with a PCR test as having HIV can be given ART. Follow your national guidelines, but in general ART should also be given to sick children under 18 months with a positive HIV antibody test if PCR tests are not available. Once a child is 18 months old, the antibody test should be repeated and ART stopped if the child does not have HIV. (If the child is still breastfeeding, wait until 3 months after breastfeeding has stopped to perform the test.) It is important to treat not just the child; the parents and other children often need ART as well and this can help the child live a healthier life.

Children under 3 years old, or under 10 kg, should be given: AZT and 3TC and NVP

Children over 3 years old and over 10 kg should be given: AZT and 3TC and EFV

DOSES FOR CHILDREN

AZT: For a child weighing:
- 5 kg to under 7 kg   give 7 ml by liquid (70 mg) 2 times a day.
- 7 kg to under 15 kg   give 100 mg 2 times a day.
- 15 kg to under 25 kg   give 200 mg 2 times a day.
- 25kg to under 40 kg   give 300 mg 2 times a day. At age 13, give adult dose.

3TC: over 30 days old   give 4 mg/kg 2 times a day. At age 16, give adult dose.

NVP:
- For children under 8 years   give 4 mg/kg once a day for 2 weeks, then give 7 mg/kg 2 times a day.
- For children 8 years and older   give 4 mg/kg 2 times a day.

EFV: For a child weighing:
- 10 to under 15 kg   give 200 mg by capsule (or 270 mg = 9 ml liquid) once a day.
- 15 to under 20 kg   give 250 mg by capsule (or 300 mg = 10 ml liquid) once a day.
- 20 to under 25 kg   give 300 mg by capsule (or 360 mg = 12 ml liquid) once a day.
- 25 to under 33 kg   give 350 mg by capsule (or 450 mg = 15 ml liquid) once a day.
- 33 to under 40 kg   give 400 mg by capsule (or 510 mg = 17 ml liquid) once a day.
- over 40 kg   give 600 mg once a day.

For second line treatments, discuss with a specialist.

Opportunistic infections

People with HIV disease have weakened immune systems. Because of this they often get opportunistic infections caused by bacteria, viruses, or fungi that do not create problems in people who are healthy. These infections are often serious and difficult to treat in people with AIDS.

Some organisms, such as *Pneumocystis jiroveci* (a fungus), cause disease only in people with weak immune systems. Other organisms, such as *Candida* (a fungus), which normally causes mild vaginal infections, can cause serious throat, vaginal, or blood infections in people with HIV. Just as each part of the world has its own animals, each part has its own opportunistic organisms: people with HIV who live in Africa will have some diseases that are the same as those of people living in Europe, and some that are different. For example, pneumonia caused by *Pneumocystis jiroveci* is rare in Africa but common in Europe.

People with AIDS often have more than one opportunistic infection. This may cause difficulty in diagnosis and treatment. As people with HIV become more ill, treatment becomes more difficult; in this case, giving medicines becomes less important than providing support and comfort (see Chapter 10). This is a time to ask your patient (and yourself) what she wants and expects from your treatment. Sometimes the best treatment will be none at all.

This appendix discusses some of the diseases seen in people with HIV and their treatments. We are trained as Western doctors and are most familiar with Western medicine, which uses X-rays, pills, and injections to diagnose and treat disease. We list several treatments for each disease based on our experience and reading. We also discuss treatments that may be necessary to prevent illnesses from returning; often these medicines must be given for the rest of a person's life. The list of diseases and treatments is not complete. In addition, many of the recommended drugs may not be available or are too expensive for most patients. In many cases there are other treatments, including local ones such as medicinal herbs or acupuncture. Most people use a combination of treatment approaches, and this appendix is meant as a framework; diagnosis and treatment should be adapted to what is available in your community. In addition, diagnosis and treatment change over time as the world learns more about HIV, and all of these recommendations should be read with this in mind.

The information in this appendix was obtained from books and articles listed in the resources section and from the authors' personal experience. The standards of care and therapies available for HIV and HIV-related illnesses are continually changing. The clinical recommendations in this book are neither absolute nor universal recommendations, and in no way supervene the informed clinical judgment of treating practitioners. The reader is advised to consult package inserts and other references before using any therapeutic agent. The authors and publisher disclaim responsibility for any adverse effects resulting directly or indirectly from omissions or undetected errors.

Skin diseases

HIV disease often causes skin problems that may not be life-threatening but can make a person miserable.

Atopic dermatitis

Atopic dermatitis begins as dry, itchy skin. Because people scratch their skin it becomes red and raised and develops scales. Atopic dermatitis is often found where the arms and legs bend. People with asthma or allergies are more likely to have atopic dermatitis than others.

Treatment:
- Avoid strong soaps or excessive bathing. These can cause dry skin and make the problem worse.
- Apply moisturizing cream 2 to 4 times a day.
- Use a steroid-containing cream or ointment like 1%–2.5% hydrocortisone cream 2 times a day.

Do not use strong steroid creams or ointments on the face or genital areas because these medicines weaken the skin.

Bacillary angiomatosis and bacillary peliosis

Bacillary angiomatosis (BA) and bacillary peliosis (BP) are diseases caused by *Bartonella henselae* or *Bartonella quintana*. These bacteria are carried by fleas and lice. They cause fragile, bright red and purple raised bumps and can

How to name skin problems		
Type of lesion	Smaller than 1 cm	Larger than 1 cm
Flat	macule	patch
Raised	papule	plaque
Fluid-filled	vesicle	blister or bulla
Pus-filled	pustule	abscess

Drug reactions

Acyclovir: Kidney damage with high IV doses if not given enough fluids; also gastrointestinal problems, headache, confusion, tremor, seizures.

Amphotericin B: Fever, chills, low potassium, low magnesium, kidney damage, low red blood cell count, vein inflammation.

Ceftriaxone: Rash, nausea, diarrhea.

Ciprofloxacin: Nausea, diarrhea, vomiting, headache, rash.

Clindamycin: Diarrhea, nausea, vomiting, rash, liver damage.

Dapsone: Methemoglobinemia, red blood cell destruction, "dapsone syndrome" (rash, fever, and liver damage, usually after 3–8 weeks of treatment), hepatitis.

Doxycycline: Nausea, diarrhea, tooth discoloration in children who receive the drug or whose mothers received it when pregnant, severe rash (avoid sunlight). Avoid in pregnancy.

Erythromycin: Nausea, vomiting, abdominal pain. IM shots are extremely painful. IV administration causes vein inflammation. Rarely, jaundice.

Ethambutol: Decreased vision, abdominal pain, rash.

Fluconazole: Nausea, vomiting, diarrhea, abdominal pain, rash. Rarely, liver damage.

Flucytosine: Low platelet count, low white blood cell count, nausea, vomiting, rash, liver damage.

Foscarnet: Kidney damage, bone marrow damage, low calcium, irregular heart rhythms, low or high phosphate, low potassium, low magnesium, low red blood cell count, penile sores.

Ganciclovir: Low white blood cell and platelet counts from bone marrow damage.

Isoniazid: Hepatitis, rash, nerve damage, nausea. Hepatitis is more common in older patients.

Ketaconazole: Nausea, vomiting, abdominal pain, liver damage.

Metronidazole: Metallic taste in mouth, nausea, abdominal pain, drowsiness. Severe abdominal pain and vomiting are common in patients who drink alcohol within two days of taking the medicine.

Penicillin: Nausea, vomiting, rash. Severe allergic reactions, such as Stevens-Johnson syndrome (a life-threatening skin reaction) and anaphylaxis, can also occur.

Primaquine: Red blood cell destruction, methemoglobinemia, low or high white blood cell count, nausea, vomiting, headache, rash.

Pyrazinamide: Hepatitis, gout.

Pyrimethamine: Abdominal pain, vomiting, tremor, rash (including Stevens-Johnson syndrome), low red blood cell count, diarrhea, vomiting, nausea.

Rifampin: Rash, nausea, vomiting, liver damage, orange urine and tears.

Sulfadiazine: Rash, kidney stones, hepatitis, low white blood cell count.

Tetracycline: Nausea, diarrhea, tooth discoloration in children who receive the drug or whose mothers received it when pregnant. Rarely, pancreatitis with large doses. Avoid in pregnancy. Sun sensitivity is common, avoid sunlight.

Thiacetazone: Rash, Stevens-Johnson syndrome.

Trimethoprim-sulfamethoxazole: Rash (including Stevens-Johnson syndrome), anaphylaxis, nausea, vomiting, low white and red blood cell counts from bone marrow damage, kidney problems, hepatitis, high potassium.

cause swollen lymph nodes, fever, and malaise. In people with HIV, Bartonella can cause serious problems of the skin, lymph nodes, lungs, heart, liver, bone, spleen, brain, digestive tract, blood, or bone marrow. It can be deadly.

BA and BP may look like Kaposi's sarcoma but lesions are usually redder and have a collar of scale around the lesion.

BA and BP can be diagnosed with a biopsy, examined with a modified silver stain such as Warthin-Stary. If available, a blood culture may be used to confirm the diagnosis.

For bacillary angiomatosis or peliosis of the skin, use erythromycin 500 mg by mouth 4 times a day, doxycycline 100 mg twice a day, or rifampin 600 mg once a day. Continue treatment for 14–21 days. If the bones or viscera are involved, treatment should continue for at least 8 weeks.

Drug reactions

Rashes are common among people using medications for opportunistic infections and HIV. These rashes are caused by reactions to medicines or combinations of medicines, especially antibiotics such as penicillin and sulfa-containing drugs. Most reactions are macular and papular eruptions, but sometimes they cause hives or the life-threatening Stevens-Johnson syndrome. Drug rashes usually start within 1–2 weeks of starting a medication. The drug or drugs suspected of causing the reaction should be stopped. The person may also need medicines to treat the reaction.

Sometimes a medicine is so important to the health of a person with HIV that it has to be used even if it causes a minor drug reaction. Try gradually increasing the dose of a medicine over several days or weeks to avoid a reaction. You can also give the person diphenhydramine 25 mg before giving the drug to prevent a reaction.

Folliculitis and eosinophilic folliculitis

Folliculitis is an infection of the skin at the root of a hair. It causes a red, itchy, or painful bump that may be filled with pus. The bumps often have a hair in the middle. Folliculitis is commonly found on the face, trunk, buttocks, and groin. Common bacteria such as *Staphylococcus aureus* or *Streptococcus* cause most cases of folliculitis. If folliculitis causes a deeper infection, a furuncle or boil (a 1–2 cm tender, red, pus-filled nodule) can occur.

Treatment:
- Soak affected areas in hot water or press a hot cloth against the area several times a day.
- Let the furuncles open themselves. Pressing or popping the boil may spread the infection. But if the furuncles do not open after 3 days, they may need to be cut open with a sterile scalpel to remove the pus.
- Apply antibiotic cream or ointment to the area.

If the person with folliculitis gets a fever give dicloxacillin 500 mg 4 times a day for 7 to 21 days.

Eosinophilic folliculitis is a type of folliculitis that consists of small red papules on the face and trunk that itch intensely. If folliculitis is not responding to the usual treatments, a biopsy can be used to look for eosinophilic folliculitis. The exact cause is not known; however, treatment with antihistamines or oral antifungal agents can be helpful.

Fungal skin infections

Many types of fungal infections cause skin problems for people with HIV. Tinea pedis causes scaling and cracks on the feet (athlete's foot). Tinea capitis causes hair loss and sores on the head. Tinea corporis causes ring-like patches on the body (ringworm); Tinea unguium infection can cause destruction of the nails; and Tinea versicolor can cause light patches on the skin. *Candida* affects the skin on moist areas of the body, such as on and around the genitals, causing redness and irritation. All can be treated with a topical antifungal cream or powder such as nystatin or miconazole.

Impetigo

Impetigo is a bacterial infection of the skin caused by *Streptococcus* and *Staphylococcus* species. The bacteria cause a red area of skin with yellow crusts, sores, and blisters; the area can be large and painful. The skin peels off easily. Impetigo may become serious if the bacteria enter the blood. Impetigo is common in children and can be easily diagnosed.

Gently soak off the crusts 3–4 times a day using soap and clean water. Paint the sores with gentian violet or another drying agent and cover with antibiotic ointment, such as bacitracin. Give dicloxacillin 500 mg by mouth 4 times a day for 7–10 days.

Itching, or prurigo

People with HIV often have skin that itches on many parts of the body. There may be small (1–2 cm), itchy papules on the skin. Itching can be treated with oral antihistamines such as hydroxyzine and diphenhydramine.

People with HIV frequently have severe reactions to insect bites, including those of mosquitoes, fleas, and flies. They should try to avoid insects by removing them from the home and by wearing insect repellent. Bites at night can be reduced by using bed netting and wearing long-sleeved shirts and long pants. Treatment for itching can include antihistamines (e.g., hydroxyzine 50–75 mg 3 times a day), or, if especially severe, topical steroid creams.

Kaposi's sarcoma

Before HIV, Kaposi's sarcoma (KS), a cancer, was usually found in men between 50 and 70 years old. It was seen on the extremities and was rarely fatal. Now most KS is found in people with HIV disease. It is caused by human herpesvirus 8 (HHV8). KS lesions are usually red, purple, or black, and are small (0.5–2 cm), firm papules and plaques. KS is often found inside the mouth, especially on the roof. The lesions can become quite large and may block lymph vessels and cause swelling of the arms or legs. KS on the soles of the feet, on the arms or legs, or in the groin may make it difficult to move. Skin cancers, moles, or bacillary angiomatosis may also look like KS; a biopsy should be done for diagnosis. KS often causes disfigurement, and people who have it may suffer from discrimination. Most people with KS have limited disease; however, severe KS can be fatal because of involvement of internal organs such as the gut or lungs.

Treatment of KS rarely lengthens life but can make a person more comfortable. There are many ways to treat KS on the skin. Most of them cause a sore that eventually heals. A cotton swab with liquid nitrogen or dry ice can be put on the KS until the bumps turn white (approximately 15 seconds). This treatment can be done every 2–3 weeks until the bumps disappear. Another treatment is vinblastine, which can be injected inside KS bumps. A small (tuberculin) syringe containing 0.01 mg of vinblastine in 0.1 ml of sterile water is used. This usually shrinks the size of the bump and may be repeated as needed. If the person has many areas that need treatment, care should be taken that the person does not get too much medicine at one time.

Radiation (800 cGy) can also be used for large areas of KS. Whole-body treatment may be necessary for people with KS over large parts of the body or in organs such as the lungs and liver: vincristine 2 mg is given once a week, vinblastine 0.5–1 mg/kg once a week by mouth, and bleomycin 10 mg/m^2 every 14 days.

Leishmaniasis

Leishmaniasis is an infection with the parasite *Leishmania* that is spread by the bite of the sandfly. The disease is more common in areas around the equator. It affects the skin and internal organs.

Skin leishmaniasis occurs about 24 months after the sandfly bite. It starts as pale bumps on the skin of the face, ears, hands, and legs; the bumps can become infected by bacteria and develop into open sores. The bumps and sores may eventually get better. Sometimes they move to the nose and throat, causing large internal sores months to years after the original sandfly bite.

Visceral leishmaniasis, or kala-azar, usually appears around 3 months after the fly bite. Symptoms include skin sores, fever, diarrhea, and cough. Internal organs such as the spleen, bone marrow, or liver may also be affected. Lymph nodes may swell.

HIV causes *Leishmania* that had been living quietly in a person's body to spread. How ill a person with HIV and leishmaniasis becomes depends on the type of *Leishmania* involved and the strength of the person's immune system. Biopsies of affected skin, bone marrow, spleen, or lymph nodes can Biopsies of affected skin, bone marrow, spleen, or lymph nodes can support the diagnosis. Cultures of the peripheral blood buffy coat may be positive. People with HIV disease may have the parasites in unusual sites, such as bronchoalveolar lavage fluid or pleural effusions. Whereas a swollen spleen is common in HIV-negative people with leishmaniasis, HIV-positive people with leishmaniasis may not have this sign.

Visceral leishmaniasis can be treated with sodium antimony gluconate 20 mg of Sb/kg once a day to a maximum daily dose of 850 mg, for 20–40 days. Amphotericin B 0.5–1 mg/kg IV every other day or pentamidine 3–4 mg/kg IV every other day for 5–25 days may also work. Skin leishmaniasis can be treated with shorter courses (around 10 days) of the same drugs. Sodium antimony gluconate, amphotericin B, and pentamidine may cause life-threatening side effects (see the box on drug reactions earlier in the appendix). Although it is difficult to escape sandflies in areas where they are endemic, people with HIV disease should be especially careful to avoid being bitten by them.

Molluscum contagiosum

Molluscum contagiosum is caused by a virus. It is seen as small, pearl-colored bumps with central dimples. The bumps are commonly found on the face, anus, and genitals. Shaving can spread the virus and the bumps. The appearance of small flesh-colored bumps with central dimpling is usually enough to make the diagnosis of molluscum.

Molluscum can be treated by applying cantharidin ointment to facial bumps. Wash off the ointment after 4–6 hrs. Do not use this on the anus or genitalia. Curettage (scraping with a sharp, curved knife), electrosurgery (burning with electricity), or carbolic acid may also be used to remove the bumps. Liquid nitrogen or dry ice, applied in small amounts for 15–30 seconds, also works well. All treatments may be repeated every 2–3 weeks until the bumps disappear.

Psoriasis

Psoriasis is a skin disease that causes red to blue-gray plaques with silvery scale and sharply defined edges. They are found mostly on the elbows, knees, and lower back. In advanced HIV disease plaques may be found in the underarms and groin. Pitting of the nails may also occur. It is not known what causes psoriasis. Treatments help, but it rarely goes away completely. It is occasionally associated with severe arthritis.

Scratching worsens psoriasis. Sunshine improves it. For psoriasis on the scalp, remove the crusts with 2–3% salicylic acid in olive oil. Then shampoo with coal tar shampoo, selenium sulfide, or zinc pyrithione. For psoriasis anywhere on the body except the face or genitals, steroid creams such as triamcinolone acetonide 0.1% or hydrocortisone 2.5% 3 times a day, or tar-based ointments 3 times a day, can be used for as long as needed (usually months or years).

Scabies

Scabies is caused by a mite that burrows into the skin. It usually digs into the areas between fingers and toes and into the armpits and groin. It causes intense itching and small red burrows. A skin scraping of a burrow, looked at under the microscope, may show a scary-looking mite. Treatment is lindane or 5% permethrin, rubbed over the entire body (except the face), washed off after 12 hours, and repeated one week later. Clothes and bedding should be washed in hot water at the same time to kill the mites.

Seborrheic dermatitis

Seborrheic dermatitis causes patches of fine, white to yellow, greasy scales on the skin. Sometimes the patches are slightly red. Seborrheic dermatitis is usually found on the scalp, eyebrows, folds of skin next to the nose and behind the ears, chest, upper back, underarms, and groin.

Seborrheic dermatitis on the scalp can be treated with a selenium sulfide–based shampoo or a ketaconazole shampoo. Hydrocortisone 1% or 2.5% cream, or other steroid-containing creams, can be applied to affected areas twice a day. Adding ketoconazole 2% cream twice a day may also help. For severe cases, in addition to the creams, give ketoconazole 200–400 mg by mouth once a day for 2–4 weeks. Topical creams may need to be used for months to years.

Shingles (herpes zoster, zona, varicella zoster)

Shingles is a painful infection of nerves in the skin caused by the chicken pox virus (varicella zoster virus, or VZV). Shingles happens when VZV, which has been living quietly inside a nerve since the time a person had chicken pox, appears again. In people with HIV, shingles can occur at any age. It is often the first sign of HIV disease.

VZV causes a patch of small, very painful vesicles and blisters, which crust over. The blisters are found in a pattern where a nerve meets the skin, and they may merge together. Shingles usually occurs on only one side (right or left) of the body, in the area where one nerve reaches the skin. The appearance of blisters in distinct patches on only one side of the body is usually enough to make a diagnosis; however, if there is any doubt, a Tzanc preparation will reveal multinucleated giant cells. VZV can sometimes spread to internal organs like the lungs; this can be fatal.

Shingles is very painful, and strong pain drugs are usually needed. The pain may continue even after the blisters are gone. Put light bandages over the rash so clothes do not rub the skin. Burow's solution or other skin treatments that dry the blisters can be useful. Acyclovir can be used, 600–800 mg by mouth 5 times a day for 7–10 days, or 30 mg/kg IV once a day. Treatment should be started as soon as possible, as it is not useful once the blisters have crusted over. If the zoster has spread widely or is near the eyes, then give acyclovir 10–12 mg/kg IV over 1 hour every 8 hours for 7–14 days. If acyclovir does not work, consider using foscarnet 40 mg/kg IV every 8 hours for as long as needed. Antibiotics that work for skin infections, such as dicloxacillin, cephalosporins, or erythromycin, can be used if the blisters become infected by bacteria.

For pain that occurs even after the zoster is gone, medicines can include phenytoin 100 mg by mouth once a day, slowly increasing to 250–300 mg a day, or carbamazepine 100 mg by mouth once a day, increasing to 400 mg once a day over 10 days.

Skin cancer

Squamous cell carcinoma is a skin cancer that starts as a hard nodule and later forms an ulcer with hardened edges. It is caused by sunlight, radiation, or cancer-causing chemicals. The cancer is more common in light-skinned people. Leukoplakia, a white plaque inside the mouth, may be the beginning of squamous cell carcinoma when it is in the mouth or on the lips of someone who has smoked or chewed tobacco. Most squamous cell cancers can be cured if found and treated early. Taking a biopsy of the affected area is the only way to be sure it is cancer.

Removing the skin cancer is the best way to treat it. Treating the site of the ulcer and the surrounding area with radiation or electrosurgery may also help kill remaining cancer cells.

Sun sensitivity

When exposed to sunlight, some people with HIV have a skin reaction that often takes the form of red plaques or blisters. This is usually because they are taking a medication, such as doxycycline or trimethoprim-sulfamethoxazole, that causes their skin to be sensitive to sunlight. Treatment includes stopping the offending drug, covering up (for example, wearing a hat and long-sleeved clothing), or using sunblock lotion.

Eye diseases

The eye is one of the first places that signs of opportunistic diseases can be found. Most of these infections cause problems in other parts of the body as well as the eye. When a person with HIV reports symptoms of eye infection, the eyes should be examined carefully because some infections cause blindness. To see diseases of the retina you will need an ophthalmoscope. Differentiating between different infections by looking at eye findings is often difficult; it may be necessary to assume that an eye problem is caused by the same disease that is affecting another part of the body. Treatment may have to be started without being sure of the diagnosis.

Conjunctivitis

Conjunctivitis is inflammation of the white part of the eye (conjunctiva), which becomes red and produces a yellowish discharge. Conjunctivitis is usually caused by viruses for which there is no treatment. These infections go away in 1–2 weeks. A thick yellow or green discharge means that the conjunctivitis is likely to be caused by bacteria. Bacterial conjunctivitis can be treated with topical antibiotic ointments or solutions. Severe pain or loss of vision can be a sign of serious infection, and an eye doctor should be consulted.

Cotton wool spots

Cotton wool spots are the most common problem in the retinas of people with HIV disease. Cotton wool spots look like bits of white wool surrounded by small retinal hemorrhages. They are caused by small blood clots in the vessels and usually go away on their own. Spots caused by cytomegalovirus (CMV; see section below) look similiar to cotton wool spots but do not go away without treatment. People with cotton wool spots usually have no symptoms.

Cytomegalovirus

Cytomegalovirus (CMV) is a common problem in people with HIV. CMV is a virus in the same family as the herpes simplex virus and varicella zoster virus (chicken pox virus). Like herpes, CMV can live for a long time in a person without causing disease. In many communities nearly everyone has CMV by the time they reach adulthood. It is spread through sex, by sharing needles, from mother to baby before birth or during breast-feeding, and by blood transfusions. CMV can affect the eyes, lungs, adrenal glands, liver, brain, spinal cord, esophagus, or gut. About one in four people with HIV disease will have life- or sight-threatening problems caused by infection with CMV.

CMV retinitis usually affects one eye and then moves to the other. People often see small spots, or "floaters," moving across their visual fields. They may also have "blind spots" and sensitivity to sunlight. Yellow and red areas that look like "cottage cheese and ketchup" (fluid and blood) can be seen on the retina during a careful eye exam with an ophthalmoscope. Retinal detachment may occur. CMV viremia may also be detected by PCR.

Treatment for CMV retinitis is ganciclovir 5 mg/kg IV infusion over 1 hour twice a day, or 2.5 mg/kg IV every 8 hours, for 14–21 days. Maintenance therapy is one-half of the induction dose or 5 mg/kg once a day for 5–7 days per week. An alternative treatment is foscarnet 60 mg/kg IV every 8 hours for 14–21 days. Oral ganciclovir can be used for maintenance therapy. Serious side effects may occur, such as neutropenia from ganciclovir and electrolyte abnormalities and kidney damage from foscarnet, so extra care must be taken when working with them. CMV is slowed by ganciclovir or foscarnet, but not stopped. Maintenance therapy should be continued for life unless the person is receiving ART.

Herpes zoster of the eye

Herpes zoster usually affects nerves to the skin. If it also attacks a nerve to the eye, it can cause blindness. Herpes zoster blisters that appear on one half of the forehead, the side of the nose, or the eyelid are especially likely to do this. They are painful and sometimes there is conjunctivitis. The cornea may be inflamed, and the iris can be involved. In severe cases or when the zoster is near the eyes, give acyclovir 10–12 mg/kg IV over 1 hour every 8 hours for 7–14 days. Acyclovir can cause renal problems and adequate hydration is necessary. If IV acyclovir is not available, it can be given 600–800 mg by mouth 5 times a day for 7–10 days. If acyclovir does not work, consider using foscarnet 40 mg/kg IV every 8 hours for as long as needed.

Kaposi's sarcoma of the eyelids

People with HIV may develop KS on their eyelids or eyes. Treatment is needed only if the KS is bothersome to the patient. Treatment may involve both local and systemic therapy (see the section on KS under "Skin diseases").

Pneumocystis jiroveci retinitis

Pneumocystis jiroveci causes multiple yellow plaques on the retina. The treatment for *Pneumocystis jiroveci* in the eye is similar to the treatment for *Pneumocystis jiroveci* pneumonia (PCP). Trimethoprim-sulfamethoxazole, pentamidine, or clindamycin are useful (see the section on PCP under "Chest diseases").

Toxoplasma chorioretinitis

Toxoplasma is a microscopic parasite spread by undercooked meat and pet cats. It causes homogenous, yellow-white, edematous retinal lesions with fluffy borders. Usually people with *Toxoplasma* have vitreitis and inflammation of the anterior segment of the eye, symptoms not seen in CMV. *Toxoplasma* lesions are not bloody. Many people with toxoplasmosis in the eye will also have it in other places, such as the brain. The treatment for *Toxoplasma* chorioretinitis is the same as the treatment for systemic toxoplasmosis (see the section on toxoplasmosis encephalitis under "Nerve and brain problems").

Nerve and brain problems

Cryptococcal meningitis

Cryptococcus neoformans is a yeast-like fungus found worldwide in soil and bird droppings. *Cryptococcus* is spread by breathing air contaminated with dust containing the fungus. (People cannot spread the fungus to each other.) The symptoms of cryptococcosis develop slowly. They include nausea, vomiting, seizures, headache, fever, and confusion. The headache is usually in the forehead above the eyes. Many people experience neck stiffness and sensitivity to light. People may also have signs of *Cryptococcus* in the lungs, kidneys, blood, prostate, and skin.

The most useful test for *Cryptococcus* is to examine the cerebrospinal fluid (CSF) for fungus, using an india ink stain and a microscope. You will see round organisms, each surrounded by a clear area. Blood and CSF can also be tested for *Cryptococcus* protein. Other studies of the CSF, such as levels of protein and glucose levels and cell counts, are often close to normal.

Severe cryptococcosis can be treated with amphotericin B 0.6–0.8 mg/kg IV per day, to a total dose of 750–1,000 mg, along with flucytosine 25 mg/kg by mouth every 6 hours, for 2 weeks followed by 8 weeks of fluconazole at

400 mg/day. For increased intracranial pressure, the patient will require daily lumbar punctures until the CSF opening pressure normalizes. Fluconazole 200–400 mg by mouth once a day can be used in mild cases for initial treatment and to prevent recurrence of symptoms. Amphotericin B is a very toxic drug and the patient should be watched closely for signs of renal failure, low magnesium, low potassium, and anemia. Flucytosine can cause myelosuppression, leading to leukopenia or a low platelet count.

Cryptococcosis will return if suppressive therapy is not given after initial treatment. Maintenance therapy is fluconazole 200 mg by mouth once a day or amphotericin B 0.5–1 mg/kg IV 1–3 times a week. Ketoconazole can also be given at 400 mg by mouth once a day. Therapy should be continued for life. If the patient starts taking ARV, they may be able to discontinue treatment after 6 months.

HIV dementia

Dementia is the most common brain problem from HIV disease. Many people with HIV will get dementia, which may cause personality changes and confusion, and may also affect coordination and mobility. People may forget things easily and lose their ability to do simple mental tasks, such as going to the market or remembering people in their families. It is often difficult to notice these changes because they happen slowly. Depression is also a common part of HIV dementia. Problems with thinking usually precede problems with movement, but over time people may develop poor balance and coordination. A tap on the tendons over the joints will cause the muscles to jump very briskly. People with serious forms of HIV dementia may not be able to talk, move, or hold in urine or feces.

Before making the diagnosis of HIV dementia, look for other causes, such as opportunistic infections, metabolic problems, drug reactions, and lymphoma. People will need support, since they will slowly lose the ability to carry out daily tasks.

Lymphoma

When lymphoma, a type of cancer, occurs in the brain, it can cause headaches, confusion, personality changes, memory loss, and difficulty walking or talking. People with lymphoma can also have difficulty swallowing and may suffer from seizures or paralysis. Lymphoma in the brain usually does not cause fever or other systemic signs of illness. Toxoplasmosis may cause problems similar to lymphoma. Both diseases cause masses in the brain that may look similar on a computed tomography (CT) scan. If there is a lesion that looks like lymphoma or toxoplasmosis on a CT scan, most people treat first for toxoplasmosis because it responds to safer medicines than does lymphoma (see the section on toxoplasmosis below).

Meningitis and encephalitis

Meningitis is an infection of the covering of the brain. It can be caused by many different organisms: bacteria, fungi, viruses, and the organisms that cause sleeping sickness and syphilis. Some common signs of meningitis are fever, a stiff neck, headache, nausea, and vomiting. Meningitis causes people to be confused or, in severe cases, comatose. Diagnosis of meningitis is best made by doing a lumbar puncture and testing the fluid that surrounds the brain.

Encephalitis is inflammation of the brain. People with encephalitis may be confused, delirious, stuporous, or comatose. They may have seizures. Encephalitis may be caused by brain abscesses, malaria, toxoplasmosis, lymphoma, *Cryptococcus*, herpes simplex virus, CMV, TB, or even HIV itself.

Mental health problems

People with HIV experience anxiety and stress. HIV disease, like other serious illnesses, can cause people to lose hope. Depression is more common among individuals with HIV compared to the general population. Look for signs of depression and suicidal thoughts in people with HIV, and treat discussions of suicide seriously. Depression can cause people to lose weight, not sleep well, lose pleasure in things, and have difficulty thinking clearly. Depression can also interfere with people's ability to take ARV medicines consistently. Antidepressant medicines or counseling can help people to feel better. Sometimes mental health problems can be confused with other illnesses. It is important consider mental health problems when trying to diagnose a nerve or brain problem in a person with HIV.

Nerve problems in the arms and legs

People with HIV commonly have nerve problems in their arms and legs. The symptoms can vary from having burning feet to experiencing so much pain that it is impossible to walk. Sometimes HIV infection leads to rapid loss of the covering of nerves, which leaves people severely weak (Guillain-Barré syndrome). People may also have nerve problems caused by poor nutrition, ARVs, or viruses such as hepatitis C or CMV.

Look for treatable causes. Nutrition can be improved and vitamins taken. Nerve problems caused by drugs can be helped by stopping or decreasing

Peripheral nerve problems in people with HIV
Distal symmetric polyneuropathy (DSPN): Tingling, burning, and pain in hands, feet, and legs. Best treatment is medicines good for nerve pain, such as tricyclic antidepressants and narcotics.
Acute and chronic inflammatory demyelinating polyneuropathy (CIDP): This is Guillain-Barré syndrome that lasts for a long time. Characterized by an increasing loss of ability to move the arms and legs, without loss of sensitivity to touch, heat, or pressure.
Mononeuritis multiplex: This is a loss of function in a single nerve. It can be seen as the inability to lift a foot or use a hand and is usually caused by CMV infection.
Cauda equina syndrome: Severe pain and weakness in the back and legs, also frequently caused by CMV.

the dose of the drug. Viruses can sometimes be treated. Otherwise, treat the person with analgesics such as aspirin, acetaminophen, tricyclic antidepressants, or narcotics.

Progressive multifocal leukoencephalopathy

Progressive multifocal leukoencephalopathy (PML) is caused by the JC virus. The virus destroys the coverings of the nerves in the brain and causes increasing weakness, difficulty swallowing, loss of vision, inability to walk, loss of memory, and difficulty thinking and speaking. There is no good treatment for PML.

Toxoplasmosis encephalitis

Toxoplasma gondii is a microscopic parasite found all over the world. It is spread by eating undercooked lamb, beef, and pork and through cat feces. About 75% of people in the world have the parasite in their bodies. Most people do not know when they have toxoplasmosis; the *toxoplasma* lives quietly within them. If the immune system is damaged by HIV, signs of toxoplasmosis begin to emerge. At first the person may have fever, a mild headache, confusion, and seizures. Some experience personality changes, signs of dementia, or problems walking or seeing. About one-third of all people who have HIV and *toxoplasma* infection will have toxoplasmosis encephalitis. *Toxoplasma* can also affect other parts of the body, including the eyes, gut, lungs, heart, and testes.

A sample of the CSF may show the organism itself (use a Wright-Giemsa stain and a microscope). Blood tests that look for antibodies against Toxoplasma cannot tell the difference between an old and a new infection, though most people with an antibody titer greater than 1:1,000 have an active infection. Although most people have already been infected with toxoplasma, those who have not may be able to avoid infection. Meat should be very well cooked (at 60 degrees centigrade for 10 minutes), smoked, or cured in brine. People should avoid touching their mouths and eyes while handling raw meat, and should wash their hands, kitchen surfaces, fruits, and vegetables thoroughly. They also should not touch cat feces.

Toxoplasmosis can be treated by first giving pyrimethamine 200 mg, followed by 50–100 mg by mouth once a day, with folinic acid 10 mg by mouth once a day and sulfadiazine 1–2 gm by mouth every 6 hours, for 4–8 weeks (depending on whether the person gets better). Clindamycin 600 mg by mouth or IV every 6 hours can be substituted for the sulfadiazine. Alternative treatments are dapsone 100 mg by mouth once a day, trimethoprim-sulfamethoxazole (trimethoprim component 5 mg/kg) by mouth or IV every 6 hours, or pyrimethamine and folinic acid as discussed above.

Once treated, people require lifelong therapy to prevent symptoms from returning. You can use pyrimethamine 25–50 mg by mouth once a day, folinic acid 5–10 mg once a day, and sulfadiazine 0.5–1 gm by mouth 4 times a day. Clindamycin 300–600 mg by mouth 4 times a day can be substituted for the sulfadiazine. Pyrimethamine-sulfadoxine 25 mg/500 mg (Fansidar), one tablet 3 times a week, can also be used in place of all of the above.

Mouth problems

People with HIV often get problems in their mouths. These can be caused by bacteria, viruses, fungi, cancers, or a lack of certain vitamins. Regular dental care is essential to prevent many of these illnesses. (For more information about HIV and problems of the mouth, see the chapter on HIV/AIDS in *Where There Is No Dentist*.)

Aphthous ulcers

Aphthous ulcers are small red bumps in the mouth or esophagus that become ulcers. They are painful and may look like herpes virus sores but are never found on the outside of the lips. The appearance of small painful ulcers inside the mouth is usually enough to make the diagnosis.

Mouth care is very important for people who have weak immune systems. These are some of the things that people can do to keep their mouths clean.

Brush teeth in the morning and at night.

Gently clean teeth every day with dental floss.

Soak false teeth in hydrogen peroxide each night.

Mouthwash for mouth pain

Swish and spit out the following mixture several times a day. Ingredients can be changed depending on what is available, and flavored liquids can be added to make the mouthwashes taste better.

Tetracycline	2 gm
Diphenhydramine hydrogen chloride syrup	240 ml
Hydrocortisone	60 mg
Nystatin	6 million units

If esophageal ulcers are present, swish and swallow the following mixture.

Diphenhydramine hydrogen chloride syrup	55 ml
Lidocaine injection 2%	10 ml
Magnesia-alumina suspension	175 ml

Medicines can be used to lessen the inflammation and pain. Examples include steroid creams, such as fluocinonide (Lidex) 0.05% ointment or benzocaine, applied to the ulcer up to 6 times a day. Decadron elixir (0.5 mg/ml) as a mouth rinse may also help. Decadron should not be swallowed. Elixirs are especially helpful when the ulcer is hard to reach, making it difficult to apply creams. Thalidomide can also be useful, given as 200 mg by mouth once a day until ulcers improve, then 100 mg by mouth 3 times a week for prevention. Thalidomide should not be used by women who are or might become pregnant while taking the drug, as it causes birth defects. The mouthwash described in the box on mouth care will also lessen pain from aphthous ulcers.

Dry mouth

In "dry mouth," which can be caused by drugs, the salivary glands fail to make enough saliva. Dry mouth makes tooth and gum disease more likely. Sucking hard candies or using artificial saliva will keep the mouth wet. Fluoride mouth rinses, toothpaste, chewing sticks, or toothpicks may help prevent cavities, which are more common in people with dry mouth.

Hairy leukoplakia

Hairy leukoplakia is a white, stuck-on–looking plaque that is usually found on the side of the tongue. The white plaques look like thrush, but unlike thrush they do not scrape off. Hairy leukoplakia generally causes no problems. The appearance is usually enough to make the diagnosis, but a biopsy can also be done to look for cancer (which can look similar), especially in people who use tobacco.

Herpes simplex virus

Herpes simplex virus (HSV) infection is very common. It is the cause of "blisters" or "cold sores" on the mouth and lips and in the genital area. Fever, sore throat, and swollen lymph nodes sometimes accompany the blisters, especially during the first outbreak. Some people feel tingling and numbness several hours before an outbreak of blisters. The painful red sores last for about two weeks in people without HIV, but in people with HIV the blisters and sores can last for many weeks. Outbreaks of blisters can occur several times in a year. Contact with the mouth or genitals of someone who has herpes can spread herpes to other people. Herpes sores also make it easier for HIV to spread from one person to another during sex. The diagnosis of herpes is usually made by recognizing the typical appearance of the sores or by examining the fluid from a blister under the microscope using a Tzanc smear.

Most cases of recurrent HSV blisters last about a week. For blisters lasting over 10 days, or for blisters in the esophagus, give acyclovir 200 mg by mouth 5 times a day or 15–30 mg/kg IV once a day. If acyclovir does not work, foscarnet 40 mg/kg IV every 8 hours for 21 days can be used.

Stress and sunlight on the face can bring out herpes blisters. For blisters that occur frequently, acyclovir 200–400 mg by mouth 2–4 times a day can be used to lower the number of attacks. This treatment can be used safely for several years.

Inflamed gums, or gingivitis

Gingivitis is an inflammation of the gums that is usually caused by bacteria. The most common signs of gingivitis are bleeding and pain in the gums after eating or brushing the teeth. Gingivitis causes the gums to pull back from the teeth. Gums may become reddened or blue. In long-standing cases the gums can be firm and light in color. These problems happen in people without HIV infection, but in people with HIV they happen more often and may be more serious. The appearance of the gums is usually enough to make the diagnosis.

People with HIV should brush their teeth or use a chewing stick every day, especially after eating sweet foods. They should use toothpaste. Toothpaste can be made by mixing salt and baking soda (bicarbonate of soda) in equal amounts. The mixture will stick to a wet toothbrush. To prevent tooth problems in children, do not bottle-feed older babies who can eat solid foods. Sucking on a bottle bathes the baby's teeth in a sweet liquid, whether milk, formula, or juice, and causes tooth decay.

For mild gum disease, remove plaque on teeth and gums with toothbrushing 2–3 times a day and use mouthwashes such as diluted hydrogen peroxide, chlorhexidine gluconate 0.2%, or povidone-iodine 10% solution.

Oral and esophageal candidiasis (thrush)

Candidiasis is caused by the fungus *Candida albicans*. *Candida* grows on areas of the body that are warm and moist, such as in the mouth, on the feet, and in the groin and vagina. It appears as white patches in the mouth and throat. It can make food taste bad and cause people to gag or have sore throats. If it is in the esophagus, it may cause difficulty swallowing. Candidiasis may appear after people take antibiotics, which kill both helpful and disease-causing bacteria living in the body, allowing the fungus to grow.

The appearance of candidiasis is usually enough to make the diagnosis. Scrape the white patch off and then spread it on a microscope slide. If it does not scrape off, it may be hairy leukoplakia (see earlier section). Add a drop or two of potassium hydroxide (KOH) solution to the scraping and then look under a microscope for the *Candida* fungi.

Treatment:

If a person has been given unnecessary antibiotics, stop them.

Gently scrub the tongue and gums with a soft toothbrush or clean cloth 3 or 4 times a day. Then rinse the mouth with salt water or lemon water and spit it out (do not swallow). In addition, use one of these remedies:

- Suck a lemon if it is not too painful. The acid slows the growth of the fungus.
- Rinse the mouth with 1% Gentian Violet liquid 2 times a day. Do not swallow.
- Put nystatin solution, 5 ml in the mouth and hold it there for 1 minute. Then swallow it. Repeat 4 times a day for 5 days.
- Dissolve nystatin tablets, 500,000 – 1,000,000 units in the mouth 3-5 times a day for 10 days or until cured.
- Dissolve clotrimazole troches, 10 mg in the mouth 5 times a day for 10 days or until cured.
- Dissolve miconazole, 250 mg in the mouth 4 times a day for 10 days or until cured.

If thrush is very bad, give ketoconazole, 200 mg by mouth 1 time a day or fluconazole 50-100 mg by mouth 1 time a day. Pregnant women should not take ketoconazole. Treatment may take months.

For candidiasis of the esophagus, take one of the following:

- Fluconazole, 100-200 mg by mouth1 time a day for 2-3 weeks.
- Ketoconazole, 200-400 mg 1 time a day for 2-3 weeks. Do not take if pregnant.

If those medicines do not work give amphotericin B 0.3 mg/kg IV 1 time a day for 7 days.

Periodontitis and necrotizing stomatitis, or "trench mouth"

Gingivitis may become the more serious periodontitis, or "trench mouth." Periodontitis is an inflammation that destroys teeth. It is a painless, quickly destructive disease that needs immediate treatment. The gums between the teeth develop ulcers and a gray look. If the gray covering is removed, a tender, bleeding area is left with a "punched out" look. The person often has a foul taste and odor in the mouth.

If treated early as gingivitis, the disease is reversible. Once periodontal disease is present, some of the gum is already lost and the person should see a dentist to smooth any rough surfaces on fillings, correct tooth position problems, and remove mobile teeth. In addition, dead tissue next to teeth may have to be removed. Mouthwashes with 0.2% chlorhexidine gluconate or 10% povidone-iodine solution will help by stopping bacteria from growing. Without treatment, periodontal disease may progress to necrotizing stomatitis, a painful disease associated with spontaneous bleeding and destruction of gingiva and bone. Treatment involves debridement, curettage, and povidone-iodine and chlorhexidine mouthwashes. Metronidazole 250 mg by mouth 4 times a day or clindamycin 300 mg by mouth 3 times a day for 5 days can be added.

Diseases of the gut

All parts of the gastrointestinal (GI) system, from the mouth to the anus, can be affected by HIV disease. Sometimes people with HIV have problems with swallowing, vomiting, diarrhea, and weight loss. These result in loss of fluids. Most people need two liters or more of fluid a day. People with diarrhea need much more.

Diarrhea

People with HIV often have severe diarrhea. To prevent infections that cause diarrhea, people should try to avoid food and water that might be contaminated. To make fresh vegetables and fruit safe, soak them for 20 minutes in 1 liter of water with 5–10 drops of bleach. If this is not possible, a good rule is to "boil it, cook it, peel it, or forget it."

Giving oral or IV fluid and treating the cause of the diarrhea can be life-saving (see the box on oral rehydration therapy). Sometimes it is impossible to tell what is causing the diarrhea. Antibiotics can be used to treat the most common infections and can be given even when the exact cause of the diarrhea is not known. Lomotil or Imodium 1–2 pills by mouth after every loose stool will often stop the diarrhea but does not treat the cause. Some people may still have 5–6 liters of diarrhea a day. For these people other treatments, such as deodorized tincture of opium 0.6 ml by mouth four times a day, or long-acting morphine sulphate 15 mg by mouth once a day, may be needed.

Salmonella and *Shigella* are more common in people with HIV than the general population. Symptoms include stomach cramping, nausea, and diarrhea, sometimes with blood and mucus. *Salmonella* can also cause a septicemia in people with HIV. These bacteria can be detected with blood and stool cultures. Give one of the following treatments. For *Salmonella* treat for 7-10 days. For septicemia, treat for 4-6 weeks.

- Ciprofloxacin 500 mg by mouth twice a day.
- Trimethoprim-sulfamethoxazole (Septra) 160 mg/800 mg by mouth twice a day or 5 mg/kg (based on trimethoprim) IV every 6 hours.
- Extended spectrum cephalosporins for salmonella septicemia.

For *Shigella*: treat mostly to shorten duration of illness and prevent spread to others. Treat with either ciprofloxacin or Trimethoprim-sulfamethoxazole according to the dose above for 3-7 days.

Campylobacter jejuni causes stomach cramping, nausea, and diarrhea, sometimes with blood and mucus. Diarrhea is often more severe and prolonged and invasive among people with more severe immunodeficiency. These bacteria can be detected with blood and stool cultures.

A mild case of *Campylobacter jejuni* does not need to be treated, but persistant cases should be. Give one of these drugs:

- Erythromycin stearate 500 mg by mouth 4 times a day for 7 days.
- Ciprofloxacin 500 mg by mouth twice a day for 7–10 days.
- Norfloxacin 400 mg by mouth twice a day for 7–10 days.

Dehydration from diarrhea has killed millions of people worldwide. Children with diarrhea are especially at risk. Before oral rehydration therapy (ORT) was developed, people with severe diarrhea either received fluids intravenously or they died. In many places IV equipment and fluids are not readily available, but an ORT solution can easily be made and used at the hospital, clinic, or home. ORT is much better than plain water, and the use of ORT to combat dehydration has saved millions of lives.

An ORT solution is made of water, salt, and sugar and is taken by mouth. The salt and sugar allow the body to absorb eight times as much water as it could if the person drank plain water alone. Clean water should be used in order not to cause new diarrheal illnesses. ORT can be made in several different ways. The essential ingredients are one teaspoon of salt and 8 teaspoons of sugar per liter of water. If available, add half a teaspoon of sodium bicarbonate (baking soda). One cup of orange juice or two bananas can also be added to replace lost potassium. When sugar is scarce, 50 grams of cereal flour from rice, maize (corn), sorghum, millet, wheat, or potato can be used.

If a person is unable to replace the amount of water he is losing from diarrhea, then he may need to be given IV fluids in a clinic or hospital.

Clostridium difficile causes acute, watery diarrhea with abdominal pain, fever, and leukocytosis. It often occurs after exposure to antibiotics. It can be diagnosed with a stool bioassay for *C. difficile cytotoxans*. Treat with metronidazole 500 mg by mouth 3 times a day for 7 days or vancomycin 500 mg by mouth 4 times a day for 7 days.

Mycobacterium avium-intracellulare complex (MAI or MAC) is treated with multiple drugs because it can quickly become resistant to a single medicine. See the section on MAC under "blood disorders".

Giardia lamblia causes watery discharge with foul-smelling stool. Occasionally, *Giardia* can be seen under the microscope wet mount of the stool. Treatment is metronidazole 500 mg by mouth 3 times a day, quinacrine 100 mg by mouth 3 times a day, or furazolidone 5 mg/kg, up to 400 mg a day. Treat for 7 days.

E. histolytica or "amoeba" can cause bloody diarrhea as well as liver and lung problems. *E. histolytica* cysts can sometimes be seen in the stool when examined under the microscope. Treat with metronidazole 750 mg by mouth 3 times a day for 5–10 days, followed by iodoquinol 650 mg by mouth 3 times a day for 20 days. Dehydroemetine 1–1.5 mg/kg IM once a day for 5 days, or emetine 1 mg/kg IM once a day for 5 days, can be substituted for metronidazole. These last two medicines can have toxic effects on the heart and they should not be used during pregnancy.

Cryptosporidium or *Isospora belli* causes watery diarrhea often with nausea, vomiting, fever, and abdominal pain. People may lose 1-3 liters of stool a day and the diarrhea can last for weeks. *Cryptosporidium* may also affect the biliary tract, causing liver and gallbladder problems. Small eggs can be seen in the stool when examined under a microscope using a modified Ziehl-Neelsen, auramine phenol, or saffranin stain. Currently, there is no good treatment for *Cryptosporidium* diarrhea. *Isospora belli* responds to trimethoprim-sulfamethoxazole 160 mg / 800 mg 4 times a day for 10 days, then twice a day for 3 weeks. The diarrhea usually stops within a few days after treatment is started.

If you do not know the cause of the diarrhea or there is blood in the stool, you can try treating it with ciprofloxacin 500 mg by mouth twice a day for 7-10 days or trimethoprim-sulfamethoxazole 160 mg/800 mg by mouth twice a day for 7-10 days. This will treat many bacterial infections. However, resistance to trimethoprim-sulfamethoxazole is common. If there is no improvement, take metronidazole 500 mg by mouth 3 times a day for 7 days. This will treat some of the parasites that might be causing diarrhea.

Esophageal diseases

People with HIV sometimes have pain or difficulty swallowing. Many diseases can cause these problems. Aphthous ulcers can occur in the mouth or esophagus. *Candida* irritates the esophagus much the same way it causes problems in the mouth. People with candidal esophagitis may have the feeling that food is sticking in the esophagus. HSV and CMV can cause painful ulcers in the esophagus, making swallowing painful. Rarely, lymphomas, Kaposi's sarcoma, and histoplasmosis also cause problems in the esophagus. If no obvious lesions are present in the mouth, endoscopy can help with diagnosis.

The treatment for candidal esophagitis is fluconazole 100–200 mg by mouth once a day or ketoconazole 200–400 mg by mouth once a day for 2–3 weeks. Patients should improve in 7–10 days. Amphotericin B 0.3 mg/kg IV once a day for 7 days may be used in severe cases where oral medicines do not work. Often fluconazole 100 mg a day or ketoconazole 200 mg a day is needed for life to prevent the esophagitis from returning.

The treatment for HSV esophagitis is acyclovir 5 mg/kg IV over 1 hour every 8 hours for 7–14 days. For less serious cases oral acyclovir 200–400 by mouth 5 times a day can be used for 7–14 days. Acyclovir 400 mg by mouth twice a day for life can be used after the initial treatment to prevent return of the problem.

The treatment for CMV esophagitis is ganciclovir 5 mg/kg IV over 1 hour twice a day for 14–21 days. An alternative is foscarnet 60 mg/kg IV every 8 hours for 14–21 days. Recurrence can be prevented by giving ganciclovir 5–6 mg/kg IV once a day 5 days a week for life or foscarnet 90–120 mg/kg IV once a day for life. Extra care must be taken when working with these drugs, since serious side effects may occur, including neutropenia with ganciclovir and kidney and electrolyte problems with foscarnet.

Liver and biliary diseases

HIV itself does not damage the liver, but many of the illnesses and treatments that are a part of HIV disease do. Pain and tenderness in the right upper part of the abdomen is often the first sign of liver disease. Liver disease should always be considered when this pain is present along with other signs that bile is not flowing well, such as jaundice (yellow eyes) caused by a high level of bilirubin in the blood, or an elevated alkaline phosphatase.

MAC is the most common opportunistic infection of the liver in HIV disease, causing fever and an enlarged liver. Hepatitis B and hepatitis C can also cause hepatitis, and alcohol abuse and some medicines such as isoniazid can cause hepatitis and increased liver enzymes in the blood.

Cholecystitis is inflammation of the gallbladder. Usually it is caused by stones in the gallbladder. In HIV disease, cholecystitis and inflammation of the liver and biliary tree happen in younger people even without gallstones. This may be due to infections with CMV or *Cryptosporidium*. The liver and gallbladder are painful and may be larger than normal. A thickened gallbladder or air in the walls are signs of gallbladder disease that may be seen using ultrasound imaging.

Rectal and anal problems

Bacterial abscesses, warts, HSV, KS, squamous cell carcinoma, CMV, *Neisseria gonorrhoeae*, and *Chlamydia* can all cause problems around and in the anus and rectum. Hemorrhoids, fissures, and abscesses may also be seen. As in other parts of the body, making a correct diagnosis is the key to finding a treatment. For example, a Tzanc preparation from an ulcer may show multinucleated giant cells consistent with HSV infection. A culture of the wound might grow *N. gonorrhoeae*.

Sinus infections (sinusitis)

Sinusitis is an inflammation of the sinuses caused by bacteria, virus, or fungi. The bacteria *Hemophilus influenzae* and *Streptococcus pneumoniae* may cause bacterial sinusitis. Sometimes more unusual bacteria like *Pseudomonas*, *Moraxella catarrhalis*, and *Enterobacter* may cause chronic sinusitis. Sinusitus can be a chronic problem in people with HIV, and weeks of antibiotic use may be needed. Signs of sinusitis include a stuffy nose, cough, headaches, pain over the sinuses, and a thick green or yellowish discharge from the nose. An X-ray may show fluid in the sinuses or thickening of the linings of the sinuses.

Treatment of bacterial sinusitis may include trimethoprim-sulfamethoxazole 160 mg / 800 mg by mouth twice a day, amoxicillin 500 mg by mouth three times a day, or doxycycline 100 mg by mouth twice a day for 10 days. For persistent infections, antibiotics with little resistance, such as ciprofloxacin 500 mg by mouth twice a day, can be used. For chronic sinusitis, treatment for 3–4 weeks is necessary. A decongestant can be used for the first 1–2 weeks to help drain the sinuses and relieve symptoms.

Chest diseases

People with HIV can get serious lung infections. A person with HIV should seek help if she becomes short of breath or has pain with breathing. In addition to treatments for specific lung diseases, there are ways to prevent illness. For example, medicine can be used to prevent *Pneumocystis jiroveci* pneumonia and tuberculosis, and vaccines can be used to prevent influenza infection.

Bacterial lung infections

Bacterial pneumonia

Bacteria pneumonias are common among people with HIV. They are commonly caused by *Streptococcus pneumoniae*, *Hemophilus influenza*, or *Staphylococcus aureus* and cause pneumonia with a fever, a cough that produces yellow-green sputum, trouble breathing, and chest pain. The lung may sound wet when listened to with a stethoscope or dull when tapped. Chest X rays usually show a solid area of infiltration in the lung that consists of fluid, cells, and bacteria; however, sometimes the pattern on the X-ray is diffuse rather than focal. Gram stains of sputum show white cells and bacteria. Blood cultures often grow bacteria.

Influenza virus causes the "flu." Infection with the virus makes it difficult to clear dirt and bacteria from the throat and lungs. This means that a person is more likely to become ill from bacteria like *S. pneumoniae*. Influenza and pneumococcal vaccines are helpful in preventing pneumonia. (Of course, vaccination does not help those who are already infected.)

Severe bacterial pneumonias may require IV treatment. Many different antibiotics can be used for bacterial pneumonia, including trimethoprim-sulfamethoxazole, which works against *Pneumococcus*, *H. influenza*, and *Moraxella*. Other useful medicines include second-generation cephalosporins, ampicillin, semi-synthetic penicillin, and aminoglycosides. Treatment is usually for 7–10 days. A macrolide antibiotic like erythromycin can be added if an atypical pneumonia such as *Mycoplasma*, *Legionella*, or *Chlamydia* is suspected.

If possible, a person with symptoms of pneumonia should be tested for TB, or if they have a CD4 < 200, for *Pneumocystis jiroveci pneumonia* (PCP).

Tuberculosis

Tuberculosis (TB) is the leading cause of death by infectious disease worldwide. In some countries as many as 50% of people are infected with TB, though most do not have the active disease. Those who have HIV infection as well as TB, however, are much more likely to become ill. Around 7–10% of people with both HIV and TB become ill with TB each year.

The PPD test

The purified protein derivative (PPD) test uses fragments of the killed tuberculosis organism to see if a person is infected with M. tuberculosis. The protein is injected under the skin. If there is a bump after 48–72 hours, the person is probably infected even if she does not have active disease. Each country has decided what size the bump has to be to indicate infection with TB (check your local guidelines).

Since people with HIV may have weakened immune systems, they may not react to the PPD test even if they are infected with M. tuberculosis. This failure to react, called anergy, means that a negative PPD test is not very useful in people with HIV disease—but a positive test is. In many areas of the world people are vaccinated with bacillus Calmette-Guérin (BCG) as children. In children, a positive PPD test may also mean prior BCG vaccination rather than TB. However, most adults with a positive PPD test are infected with M. tuberculosis, even if they had a BCG vaccination as a child. Persons with HIV infection who have a positive PPD and no signs of active tuberculosis can take isoniazid (INH) 300 mg by mouth once a day for 9 months to prevent the occurrence of active TB. Pyridoxine 10 mg by mouth once a day can be added to prevent nerve problems, which can result from INH treatment.

TB, which is caused by *Mycobacterium tuberculosis*, is most commonly found in the lungs but can also affect the brain, adrenal glands, kidneys, bones, gut, and blood. People with HIV are more likely to have TB outside of the lungs than people who do not have HIV. Anyone with a chronic cough, fever, weight loss, or night sweats should be examined for TB.

The diagnosis of tuberculosis is made by looking at sputum under a microscope with an acid-fast stain. If no tuberculosis bacteria are seen in three separate sputum samples, it is unlikely that the person has active tuberculosis in her lungs. Samples of sputum, urine, blood, lymph node, bone marrow, or even liver tissue can also be cultured for *M. tuberculosis*. Culture can sometimes detect *M. tuberculosis* in samples that are not positive on acid-fast stain.

People with HIV disease who have signs of TB should be treated with medicine (see below). People with HIV who have no signs of TB but are PPD-test positive (check your local guidelines for the definition of a positive test) should get at least a year of the drug isoniazid (INH) as prophylaxis (a maximum of 300 mg by mouth once a day), along with pyridoxine (vitamin B6) 10 mg by mouth once a day to prevent nerve problems.

Treatment for TB takes months or years. People with active TB should be supported so that they finish a full course of treatment. Often the clinical signs go away within a few weeks of treatment, and people may think that they are cured. If they stop treatment they risk developing drug-resistant TB, which is almost impossible to cure and can be spread to others.

Standard treatment is the following (may vary by country):

Months 1–2

isoniazid (INH) 300 mg by mouth once a day

rifampin 600 mg once a day (450 mg if weight is less than 50 kg)

pyrazinamide 25 mg/kg by mouth once a day

ethambutol 25 mg/kg by mouth once a day if extra-pulmonary disease or INH resistance is suspected

Months 3–6

INH 300 mg by mouth once a day

rifampin 600 mg by mouth once a day or 3 times a week

Prophylaxis

INH 5 mg/kg once a day (maximum dose 300 mg) for 9 months, with pyridoxine (vitamin B6) 10 mg by mouth once a day to prevent nerve problems

---

Preventing drug resistance

The spread of HIV has caused a rise in the number of people with tuberculosis. Because of this, there has also been an increase in cases of drug-resistant tuberculosis. While some people are originally infected with a drug-resistant strain of M. tuberculosis, most cases of drug resistance occur in people with tuberculosis who are given the wrong medicine, are not given treatment for the necessary amount of time, or do not take the medicine regularly. To prevent drug resistance, make sure that each person with active TB gets the right treatment for the full amount of time. Watch her take her medicines.

Fungal lung infections

Fungi are found in soil everywhere in the world. Fungi that people come in contact with can cause disease, especially if the immune system is weak. Many parts of the body, including the lungs, can be affected. Some common fungal infections of the lungs are histoplasmosis, blastomycosis, cryptococcosis, and coccidioidomycosis.

Coccidioidomycosis

Coccidioides is a fungus that causes lung infection. It is found mostly in Latin America and the southwestern United States. Most people who become sick with *Coccidioides* were infected much earlier. It often lives in healthy people without causing harm. The new illness is usually a reactivation of this old infection. Active *Coccidioides* infection causes cough, fever, weight loss, and breathing problems. A chest X ray may show small round masses in one or both lungs or enlarged hilar lymph nodes. Diagnosis can be made by doing laboratory studies on blood, sputum, and CSF. Bronchoalveolar lavage fluid stained with a periodic acid–Schiff stain may also be done to find *Coccidioides*. Biopsies of bone marrow, liver, lungs, or skin can also be useful.

Coccidioides is treated with amphotericin B 0.5–1 mg/kg IV once a day until symptoms go away (usually 6–8 weeks). Alternative treatment is fluconazole 400–800 mg by mouth once a day, ketoconazole 400 mg by mouth once a day, or itraconazole 800 mg by mouth twice a day. To prevent return of the *Coccidioides*, itraconazole 200 mg by mouth twice a day or fluconazole 400 mg by mouth once a day. Amphotericin B 1 mg/kg IV once a week for life can also be used for prevention.

Histoplasmosis

Histoplasma is a fungus found mostly in the United States, the Caribbean, and Latin America. Anybody who lives in or travels to these areas can get histoplasmosis by breathing dust that contains the organism. Histoplasmosis causes fever, weight loss, and what may look like bacterial pneumonia on a chest X ray. Diagnosis of histoplasmosis is difficult. Biopsies of bone marrow, lymph nodes, liver, and lung can be stained using a Wright-Giemsa or methenamine silver stain and examined under the microscope for the fungus. The peripheral blood buffy coat may also have the fungus. Blood and CSF can also be cultured. For histoplasmosis that has spread throughout the body, the fungus can be detected in the blood or urine.

Treatment for severe cases is amphotericin B 0.5–1 mg/kg IV once a day until symptoms go away (usually 3-10 days), followed by oral therapy with itraconazole or ketoconazole. Give itraconazole 300 mg by mouth twice a day for 3 days, then 200 mg twice a day for 12 weeks, or fluconazole 400 mg by mouth twice a day for 12 weeks. To prevent return of the histoplasmosis, itraconazole 200 mg once a day by mouth or amphotericin B 1 mg/kg IV once a week for life can be used.

Pneumocystis jiroveci pneumonia (PCP)

Pneumocystis jiroveci pneumonia (PCP) is an infection of the lungs by a small fungus called *Pneumocystis jiroveci*. It is more commonly found in Western industrialized countries than in Africa. Like *Coccidioides*, *Pneumocystis jiroveci* is found in many people's lungs but only becomes a problem when the immune system is weakened. People with PCP experience shortness of breath,

---

Trimethoprim-sulfamethoxazole desensitization

In areas of the world where PCP is common, preventing PCP in people with HIV is very important. This is true even for people with allergies to sulfa-containing medicines. You can desensitize people to trimethoprim-sulfamethoxazole by giving it in low doses and slowly increasing the amount over time. This often allows people to take this medicine safely.

Increasing dosages of trimethoprim-sulfamethoxazole elixir can be given as follows (1 teaspoon = 5 ml = 80 drops):

   1/8 teaspoon once a day for 5 days

   1/4 teaspoon once a day for 5 days

   1/2 teaspoon once a day for 5 days

   1 teaspoon once a day for 5 days

   2 teaspoons once a day for 5 days

   PCP prophylaxis: Septra DS one tablet once every day

Stop treatment if serious rash appears.

For adults, or children who can take pills, equivalent doses to those listed above can be given by splitting trimethoprim-sulfamethoxazole pills into parts.

---

fever, tiredness, weight loss, and a cough that brings up white sputum or none at all. They may have a "catch" in the chest when they take a deep breath.

PCP can be treated with one of the following: trimethoprim-sulfamethoxazole, 2 double-strength (160 mg / 800 mg) tablets by mouth three times a day, or 5 mg/kg (based on trimethoprim) IV every 8 hours, for 21 days; pentamidine 3–4 mg/kg IV mixed in 250 ml of 5% dextrose in water and given over 1 hour once a day for 21 days; dapsone 100 mg by mouth once a day for 21 days with trimethoprim 5 mg/kg by mouth every 6 hours; primaquine 15 mg base by mouth once a day for 21 days with clindamycin 600 mg IV every 6 hours; or trimetrexate 30–45 mg/m^2 IV once a day for 21 days with folinic acid 20 mg/m^2 by mouth or IV every 6 hours. Each of these treatments has significant side effects. Talk to a local pharmacist to better understand these effects. For people with moderate to severe symptoms, the addition of steroids to the antibiotic regimen can be lifesaving. Prednisone is given 40 mg by mouth twice a day for days 1–5, 20 mg by mouth twice a day for days 6–10, and 20 mg by mouth once a day for days 11–21.

People with HIV who have shown signs of having weak immune systems, including having had PCP or having been diagnosed with AIDS, should receive medicines to prevent PCP. Prophylactic treatment is trimethoprim-sulfamethoxazole 160 mg / 800 mg by mouth once every day. Pyramethamine-sulfadoxine 25 mg / 500 mg (Fansidar) can also be used, one tablet by mouth once a week. If someone is allergic to trimethoprim-sulfamethoxazole, dapsone can be given, 50–100 mg by mouth once a day for life or until ART has brought the person's CD4 count up to 200 or more for 3-6 months.

Blood disorders

Anemia

Infections, malnutrition, and drugs can cause blood disorders in people with HIV. Infections of the bone marrow can cause people to become anemic (to have a low red blood cell count), leukopenic (to have a low white blood cell count), thrombocytopenic (to have a low platelet count), or pancytopenic (to have low counts of all cell types). People with HIV and weak immune systems almost always have a mild anemia related to the disease. Other common causes of anemia are organisms like malaria and MAC; TB; and fungi, such as *Histoplasma*. Sometimes anemia is the result of kidney disease or a lack of vitamins or iron. Other causes include blood loss or destruction of the red cells. HIV also causes some white cells (CD4 cells) and neutrophils to be destroyed, which makes it difficult for people to fight common diseases.

Mycobacterium avium-intracellulare complex (MAC)

The bacteria that cause MAC are similar to *M. tuberculosis*. They are found in the soil and water in most of the world. It is not known how MAC is spread. MAC infection can cause fever, weakness, weight loss, abdominal pain, long-lasting diarrhea, and low numbers of red and white blood cells. People with advanced HIV disease are at increased risk for MAC.

MAC is diagnosed through special blood cultures or a tissue biopsy. MAC is not easy to treat and requires lifelong therapy. You can try rifampin 600 mg by mouth once a day, ethambutol 15–25 mg/kg by mouth once a day, and, if available, ciprofloxacin 500–750 mg by mouth twice a day. Amikacin can be added at a dose of 7.5 mg/kg IV or IM once a day. In the United States, either clarithromycin 500 mg by mouth twice a day or azithromycin 500–1,000 mg once a day is used with one of the following: ethambutol 15–25 mg/kg once a day, rifabutin 600 mg once a day, or ciprofloxacin 500–750 mg by mouth twice a day. Amikacin can be added at 7.5 mg/kg once a day. Rifabutin 300 mg once a day, clarithromycin 500 mg by mouth twice a day, or azithromycin 500 mg 3 times a week for life can be used to help prevent someone with severe HIV disease from getting MAC.

Sexually transmitted diseases

Sexually transmitted diseases (STDs) are very widespread, and many have become resistant to common medicines. Sexually transmitted diseases greatly increase the chance that HIV will be spread during sex (see box on treating STDs). They last longer and can be more serious in people with HIV. For these reasons, it is very important to treat sexually transmitted diseases in people with HIV. Do not forget to treat the sexual partners of your patients as well! Otherwise, the infection will return.

Chancroid

Chancroid is caused by infection with the bacteria *Hemophilus ducreyi*. It causes very tender sores (chancres) and swollen lymph nodes in the genital area. The chancres appear 1–8 days after sex with an infected partner. A diagnosis can be made by swabbing the edge of a chancre and culturing the swab for *H. ducreyi*.

Treatment is one of the following: erythromycin 500 mg by mouth 3 times a day for 7 days (in the presence of severe GI upset, decrease the dosage to 250 mg 3 times a day for 14 days); ciprofloxacin 500 mg by mouth

Men with HIV who have other STDs shed up to ten times as much HIV in their semen as men with no STDs. The more virus in the semen, the more likely that HIV will be spread. Treating the men for the STDs—such as gonorrhea, chlamydia, and trichomoniasis—drops the amount of HIV in their semen to the level of men without STDs. Treating STDs in women probably has the same effect on the level of HIV in vaginal secretions. In addition, people with STDs are much more likely to become infected with HIV during sex than people without STDs. This means that treating people for STDs is a critical tool in stopping the spread of HIV.

once; ceftriaxone 250 mg IM once; or spectinomycin 2 gm IM once. Longer treatment courses are often necessary in patients with HIV. If dark-field microscopy and blood tests for syphilis are not available, the patient should also be treated for syphilis.

Chlamydia

Chlamydia trachomatis is a sexually transmitted bacterium. Most men and women with *Chlamydia* infections do not have symptoms. However, some men may have pain with urination or a clear fluid from the penis, and in some women the cervix may be tender and produce pus. A smear of urethral or cervical fluid usually shows many white blood cells and epithelial cells but no yeasts or other organisms. A culture, however, will show *Chlamydia*.

Chlamydia infections of the urethra, cervix, eye, or rectum should be treated with doxycycline 100 mg by mouth twice a day for 7 days, or tetracycline 500 mg by mouth 4 times a day for 7 days. If the infection does not respond to doxycycline, try erythromycin 500 mg by mouth 4 times a day for 7 days, or ofloxacin 300 mg by mouth twice a day for 7 days.

Doxycycline and other tetracyclines should not be used for pregnant women. Instead, use one of the following: erythromycin 500 mg by mouth 4 times a day for 7 days; amoxicillin 500 mg by mouth 3 times a day for 10 days; clindamycin 450 mg by mouth 4 times a day for 10 days; or sulfasoxazole (or other equivalent sulfonamide) 500 mg by mouth 4 times a day for 10 days.

Infection during pregnancy can cause early delivery, low birth weight, and death of the infant. Chlamydia and gonorrhea often occur together, and all infants should be given eyedrops at birth to treat possible *N. gonorrhoeae* infection (see section below). If an infant has conjunctivitis and it does not improve immediately, erythromycin syrup 50 mg/kg should be given by mouth 4 times a week for 2 weeks to treat possible *Chlamydia* infection.

Genital herpes

Genital herpes is caused by a sexually transmitted herpes virus. Symptoms are usually most severe when a person is first infected; within a week of infection, people usually get extremely painful vesicles on the penis or vaginal lips and in the vagina and rectum. The vesicles open, crust over, and go away. However, the virus lives inside nerves and will often return, causing painful vesicles three to four times a year for the rest of a person's life. In people with HIV, these attacks can be particularly severe.

There is no cure for genital herpes. People are especially infectious to their sexual partners when the sores are present and should not have sex during these times. Treatment involves pain medicine, and if available, acyclovir. Mild attacks can be treated with acyclovir 200 mg by mouth 5 times a day for 10 days. Severe attacks can be treated with acyclovir 5 mg/kg IV every 8 hours for 5 days or until resolution of symptoms. Sores can be prevented from returning, or at least made less frequent and less severe, by giving acyclovir 400 mg by mouth 2 times a day. Foscarnet 40 mg/kg IV 3 times a day can be used for genital herpes that does not respond to acyclovir.

Gonorrhea

Gonorrhea is caused by the bacterium *Neisseria gonorrhoeae*. In women, there are often no signs of gonorrhea. Even if a woman has no symptoms, she can give the disease to others during sex or during birth. Men with gonorrhea usually have drops of white pus from the penis and pain when they urinate. In men, signs of gonorrhea usually begin 2–5 days after having sex with a person with gonorrhea. In both men and women it can cause pharyngitis after oral sex, as well as severe arthritis.

The diagnosis in men can usually be confirmed by examining discharge from the penis under a microscope and looking for *N. gonorrhoeae* inside white blood cells with a Gram stain. In women a Gram stain of cervical or urethral discharge may be positive. Fluid from men and women can also be cultured on chocolate agar for *N. gonorrhoeae*.

In many parts of the world, common medicines like penicillin, doxycycline, and tetracycline do not work against *N. gonorrhoeae* because the bacterium has become resistant to these drugs. If laboratory tests in your area have shown that one of these drugs still works, you can use it—for example, doxycycline 100 mg by mouth twice a day for 7 days. If you do not know whether any of them still work, or you know that where you live they do not work, then genital, anal, or pharyngeal gonorrhea can be treated with one shot of ceftriaxone 125–250 mg IM. Alternatives are cefixime 400 mg by mouth once; ciprofloxacin 500 mg by mouth once; ofloxacin 400 mg by mouth once; or one shot of spectinomycin 2 gm IM (this is not effective for pharyngeal infection). Trimethoprim-sulfamethoxazole 400 mg / 80 mg, 10 tablets (or 5 double-strength tablets) by mouth once a day for 3 days, can also be used, although *N. gonorrhoeae* is becoming resistant to this medicine. Anyone with gonorrhea should also be treated for *Chlamydia* infection, because they frequently occur together.

Bacteremia and arthritis can be treated with ceftriaxone 1 gm IV once a day for 7–10 days. An alternative is ceftizoxime or cefotaxime 1 gm IV every 8 hours for 2–3 days or until the person's condition improves, followed by cefixime 400 mg by mouth twice a day or ciprofloxacin 500 mg by mouth twice a day to complete 7–10 days of total therapy. In areas where these medicines still work, you can give amoxicillin 500 mg by mouth 4 times a day, doxycycline 100 mg by mouth twice a day, or tetracycline 500 mg by mouth 4 times a day, for 7–10 days.

Gonococcal conjunctivitis is treated with one of the following: ceftriaxone 125 mg IM once, plus saline washes; cefotaxime 25 mg/kg IV or IM every 8–12 hours for 7 days, plus saline washes; or penicillin G 100,000 units/kg IV each day, in 4 doses, for 7 days, plus saline washes. Neonatal meningitis is treated with cefotaxime 50 mg/kg IV every 8–12 hours for 10–14 days, or penicillin G 100,000 units/kg IV each day, in 3 or 4 doses, for at least 10 days. Urogenital, rectal, and pharyngeal gonorrhea in children weighing less than 45 kg can be treated with ceftriaxone 125 mg IM once.

The eyes of all newborn babies should be protected from gonorrhea (and possible blindness) by using 1% tetracycline ointment, 1% erythromycin ointment, or 1% silver nitrate drops at birth. This should be done even if the mother and father do not have signs of gonorrhea.

Granuloma inguinale

Granuloma inguinale is a disease caused by *Calymmatobacterium granulomatis*. It occurs in the tropics and subtropics. A papule appears in the genital area 9–90 days after sex with an infected partner. The papule becomes a painless ulcer and grows. The infection may spread from the skin to the liver, spleen, and bone. Severe scarring can occur.

Granuloma inguinale can be treated with trimethoprim-sulfamethoxazole 80 mg / 400 mg two tablets twice a day, tetracycline 500 mg by mouth 4 times a day for 14 days, chloramphenicol 500 mg by mouth 4 times a day for 21 days, or gentamicin 1 mg/kg IM 3 times a day for 21 days.

Human papillomavirus (HPV)

Human papillomavirus is a common virus that can cause warts on the penis, scrotum, vagina, vaginal walls, cervix, or anus. The virus is the leading cause of cervical cancer. About 500,000 cases of cervical cancer happen each year, 75% of them in parts of the world where screening for cervical cancer is rare. In some areas, cervical cancer is the leading cause of cancer deaths in women. Among women with HPV, those who also have HIV are more likely to get cervical cancer than those without HIV. By treating HPV, you will help prevent the spread of the virus and the cancer. Screening with Pap smears and treating women can save lives.

Warts are hard to cure and often return; treatment may need to be repeated several times. Putting vinegar or low-strength acetic acid on the warts will turn them white and help with diagnosis. Since HPV can cause cervical cancer in women after many years, it is important not only to treat the HPV, but also to closely watch women who have had it. This can be done with frequent Pap smears. Every woman with HIV should have a Pap smear done every 6 to 12 months to look for the beginnings of cancer (cervical dysplasia).

Podophyllum resin (10–25% in tincture of benzoin) or podophyllotoxin 0.5% can be used to get rid of the warts. Either should be applied to the warts once a week; the treatment may be used up to four times. Podophyllum should be placed carefully only on the warts and should be allowed to dry before coming into contact with normal skin, as it is very caustic and painful to the patient. Podophyllotoxin is less toxic and can be applied by patients themselves. Both should be washed off after 1–4 hours. Cryotherapy (frozen carbon dioxide or liquid nitrogen), immunologic therapy with aldara, and laser treatments also work well when available. Swabs should be used on only one patient and then thrown away to avoid spreading HPV to others.

Lymphogranuloma venereum (LGV)

Lymphogranuloma venereum is a *Chlamydia* infection spread through sex. The types of *Chlamydia* that cause LGV are different from the types that cause common *Chlamydia* infections. The first sign of LGV in men is a painless ulcer on the penis; in women the ulcer is usually not noticed. The ulcer heals within a few days. After a few more days to months, lymph nodes begin to swell on one side of the groin. They become painful, open sores and drain pus. There may also be painful, oozing, or bleeding sores around the anus. Other common signs are fever, fatigue, headache, and joint pain. Do not biopsy the sore, since biopsy sites do not heal well. However, LGV can cause strictures and fistulae that may require surgery despite possible problems with wound healing.

Treatment is one of the following: doxycycline 100 mg by mouth twice a day for 21 days; tetracycline 500 mg by mouth 4 times a day for 14 days; erythromycin 500 mg by mouth 4 times a day for 21 days; or sulfadiazine 1 gm by mouth 4 times a day for 14 days. Patients should avoid all sexual contact until the sores are healed, as the infection is easily spread.

Pelvic inflammatory disease (PID)

Pelvic inflammatory disease is an infection of a woman's fallopian tubes, uterus, and areas around them. The infection is sexually transmitted and is usually caused by *N. gonorrhoeae*, *Chlamydia*, or other bacteria. PID is more common and may be more serious in women with advanced HIV disease. PID can lead to severe problems such as sterility, long-term pain, and ectopic pregnancy. Ectopic pregnancies often occur in the fallopian tubes, which can rupture and cause life-threatening bleeding and infection. Women with PID usually have pelvic pain, inflammation of the cervix, or tenderness with movement of the cervix on pelvic exam. They may have an increased white blood cell count and an increased erythrocyte sedimentation rate (ESR). A pregnancy test can be used to see if a woman with PID is pregnant. If she is, an ultrasound of the pelvis can look for a pregnancy or abscess in the fallopian tubes. Surgery is necessary to treat ectopic pregnancies. If the pregnancy test is not positive, she can be treated for PID without surgery.

If a woman has an intrauterine device (IUD) in place to prevent pregnancy, it should be removed or the infection will be much more difficult to treat. Women who are not hospitalized can be treated for possible *N. gonorrhoeae* infection with cefoxitin 2 gm IM once plus probenecid 1 gm by mouth once, or ceftriaxone 250 mg IM once. Either of these treatments should be followed with doxycycline 100 mg by mouth twice a day, or tetracyline 500 mg by mouth 4 times a day, for 10–14 days to treat *Chlamydia*. To make sure most of the possible causes of PID are treated, some people also add metronidazole 500 mg by mouth 3 times a day for 10 days to treat infections by anaerobic bacteria.

Ill patients who need to stay in the hospital can be given ceftriaxone 250 mg IM twice a day for 4 days, along with doxycycline 100 mg by mouth or IV twice a day for 10–14 days. Another treatment is ciprofloxacin 500 mg by mouth twice a day, doxycycline 100 mg by mouth twice a day, and metronidazole 500 mg by mouth twice a day, for 4 days, and then doxycycline 100 mg by mouth twice a day for an additional 6–10 days. Severely ill patients should receive gentamicin 1.5 mg/kg IV every 8 hours and clindamycin 900 mg by mouth 3 times a day for at least 4 days, followed by doxycycline or tetracycline for 10 days.

Syphilis

Syphilis is caused by the bacterium *Treponema pallidum*, which is almost always spread through sex. Occasionally syphilis can be spread from a pregnant woman to her fetus or through blood transfusions. Syphilis has three stages. The first stage occurs 2–12 weeks after a person has sex with someone who has syphilis. A *painless* sore, or chancre, appears on the penis or in the mouth, vagina, or anus. It can look like a pimple, a blister, or an open sore. Syphilis chancres are infectious and can easily spread the disease. The sore heals on its own, but the bacteria are still in the person's body.

The second stage of syphilis happens weeks to months after a person is first infected. Someone with second-stage syphilis may get a sore throat, fever, mouth sores, swollen joints and lymph nodes, eye problems, inflammation of the meninges, or a skin rash. The rash is usually painful or itchy, with macules and papules on the trunk, palms, and bottoms of the feet. These skin signs, just like the first sore, will often go away by themselves, but the person still has syphilis.

The third stage of syphilis occurs months to years after the second stage. *Treponema pallidum* infects many organs and can cause stroke, meningitis, heart disease, paralysis, insanity, and death. People with HIV can have unusual forms of syphilis disease, including eye problems (retinitis, uveitis, and optic neuritis), hearing loss, and quick changes from one stage of syphilis to the next.

Syphilis can be diagnosed by using dark-field microscopy to look for *Treponema* in samples from a chancre or tissue biopsy. This is especially useful during the first or second stages, when skin lesions are often present. Blood tests for syphilis are also available: the rapid plasma reagin test (RPR), the venereal disease research laboratory (VDRL) test, and specific treponemal tests (fluorescent antibody absorbed test [FTA-Abs] and hemagglutination assays [MHA-TP, TPHA]). They do not become positive for at least two weeks after the chancre appears. RPR and VDRL are usually used as screening tests. People with HIV who have neurologic symptoms, have had syphilis for over one year, or who are having a lumbar puncture for another reason should be checked for neurosyphilis by testing CSF with a VDRL. Sometimes serum RPR and VDRL tests are positive even if the person does not have syphilis. This is called a false positive. A treponemal test can be used to be sure of the diagnosis. The treponemal tests are important in people with HIV, who have a higher chance of having a false-positive RPR than people without HIV.

With good treatment, VDRL and RPR results may become negative within a year. The treponemal tests usually remain positive for life, even if a person has been treated for syphilis, although a titer of 1:4 or less probably means the person is currently infected and should be treated. If a person who has been treated for syphilis in the past has a fourfold increase in the titer of VDRL or RPR or has had sexual contact with someone who has syphilis, then she should be re-treated for syphilis.

Pregnant women should be tested for syphilis by VDRL or RPR, and women who test positive should be treated. This not only cures them, but prevents spread of the infection to the fetus. As with other STDs, if someone has syphilis, all of her or his sexual partners should be tested and treated. This will prevent new infections in your patient as well as curing the sexual partners of a serious disease.

Treatment for the first and second stages of syphilis differs from treatment for the third.

First and second stages: Benzathine penicillin G 2.4 million units IM, usually split in two and given as two shots at different sites because of the large volume of fluid. Alternatives that have not been well tested are doxycycline 100 mg by mouth twice a day for 14 days or erythromycin 500 mg by mouth 4 times a day for 14 days.

Third stage with a normal CSF examination (latent syphilis): Benzathine penicillin G 2.4 million units IM once a week for 3 weeks, or procaine penicillin G 1.2 million units IM once a day for 3 weeks. Alternative treatments are doxycycline 100 mg by mouth twice a day for 28 days, or tetracycline 500 mg by mouth four times a day for 28 days.

Any stage with neurologic symptoms or an abnormal CSF examination: Aqueous crystalline penicillin G 3–4 million units IV every 4 hours for 14 days; or aqueous procaine penicillin G 2.4 million units IM once a day for 14 days and probenecid 500 mg by mouth 4 times a day for 10–14 days, followed by one shot of benzathine penicillin G 2.4 million units IM.

Alternative regimens for patients with neurologic symptoms: Amoxicillin 2 gm by mouth twice a day and probenecid 500 mg by mouth 3 times a day for 14 days; doxycycline 200 mg by mouth twice a day for 21 days; ceftriazone 1 gm IM once a day for 5–14 days; or benzathine penicillin G 2.4 million units IM once a week and doxycycline 200 mg by mouth twice a day, both for 3 weeks. Some doctors recommend using higher doses and longer treatments for people with HIV than for others.

Treatment of infants: Infants with syphilis should be given at least one shot of benzathine penicillin G 50,000 units/kg IM (maximum 2.4 million units). If the CSF is abnormal, then benzathine penicillin G or procaine penicillin G 50,000 units/kg should be given IM or IV once a day for 10 days. Some doctors recommend this longer 10-day course for all infants with syphilis.

Vaginal infections

A small amount of vaginal discharge or fluid is normal. The amount and character of the discharge normally changes during the month and also during a woman's lifetime. Most of the time the discharge is clear or slightly milky and has a mild odor. Women with a vaginal infection may have itching and a discharge with an unusual or bad smell.

Bacterial vaginosis

Bacterial vaginosis is the growth of bacteria that cause vaginal discharge and odor. The vaginal fluid is less acidic than normal (with a pH greater than 4.5); a sample of it will give off a fishy odor when a drop of 5–10% potassium hydroxide is added. The cause of vaginosis is not known, but the bacteria *Gardnerella vaginalis* and *Mycoplasma hominis* are suspected to play a role. A sample of the vaginal discharge viewed under the microscope may reveal "clue cells," white blood cells that are coated with bacteria.

Bacterial vaginosis can be treated with metronidazole 2 gm by mouth once, or 500 mg by mouth twice a day for 7 days, or with clindamycin 300 mg by mouth twice a day for 7 days. Ideally, treatment should be avoided during pregnancy. However, if the symptoms are severe, the 2 gm dose of metronidazole may be given after the first trimester. People taking metronidazole should not drink alcohol because it will cause vomiting and abdominal pain. Sexual partners need not be treated, as bacterial vaginosis is not spread sexually.

Trichomoniasis

Trichomonas vaginalis, a parasite, causes vaginal and penile infections. Women and men may have no symptoms yet still spread the infection through sex. In women, *Trichomonas* causes itching and a thin, foamy, greenish-yellow, foul-smelling vaginal discharge. Women often feel itching and burning when trying to urinate. Sometimes the vagina becomes red and sore. Men usually have no symptoms. An exam of the vaginal fluid or urethral discharge mixed with a drop of saline under the microscope shows small, swimming *Trichomonas* organisms.

Metronidazole 2 gm by mouth once, or 500 mg by mouth twice a day for 7 days, can be used to treat trichomoniasis. As with bacterial vaginosis, treatment should ideally be avoided during pregnancy. However, if the symptoms are severe, a single 2 gm dose of metronidazole may be given after the first trimester. People taking metronidazole should not drink alcohol because it will cause vomiting and abdominal pain. Sexual partners need to be treated as well, or the infection will return.

Trichomonas infects infants at the time of birth and usually goes away in a few weeks without treatment. If an infection remains 4 weeks after birth, give metronidazole 5 mg/kg by mouth 3 times a day for 5 days.

Vaginal candidiasis

Vaginal candidiasis, or yeast infection, is a common problem in women. It is caused by the fungus *Candida albicans*, which also causes oral thrush. It is especially common in women with HIV and is often the first HIV-related disease in women. Women who have frequent candidiasis, or infections that do not get better with treatment, should consider having an HIV test.

Candidiasis causes the vaginal wall to be covered by a thick, white, creamy fluid. When the white patch is scraped off it leaves a red, irritated area behind. *Candida* grows more rapidly when the vagina is free of bacteria, when it has less acid, or when there is a lot of sugar in the blood (such as in people with diabetes). Frequently, women taking antibiotics will get yeast infections; antibiotics kill both bad and good bacteria, leaving more room for the fungus to grow rapidly. Yeast infections are also common during menses and pregnancy, and after douching.

You can test for candida by adding a drop of 5–10% potassium hydroxide solution to a sample of the vaginal fluid. Then look under a microscope for spores and branches of yeast.

It may be difficult to treat a yeast infection while a woman is taking antibiotics. Topical butoconazole, clotrimazole, miconazole, nystatin, terconazole, or tioconazole cream or suppositories can be used for 3–7 days to clear the fungus. Sometimes treatment for up to 2 weeks is needed. In severe cases, ketoconazole 150 mg by mouth once, fluconazole 150 by mouth once, or itraconazole 200 mg by mouth once can be used. They are very effective but expensive. Sometimes medicines need to be given regularly for months to prevent infections from returning.

HIV and pregnancy

Women with HIV but no symptoms have no more difficulty with pregnancy than other women. However, opportunistic infection and some medicines used to treat them can affect a fetus. For this reason, infections in pregnant women are often difficult to treat. The health of both the fetus and the mother must be taken into account before giving a pregnant mother medicines. In some cases it may be best not to treat an infection.

Pregnant women with HIV will be confronted with several decisions. You can guide them through some of the most difficult ones.

Counseling about reproductive choices. This includes discussing ways to avoid unplanned pregnancies. Abortion may be an option for women who decide that they do not want to have a child or take the risk of having a child with HIV.

Testing. Tests for syphilis, gonorrhea, chlamydia, hepatitis B, and TB are a good idea for pregnant women with HIV.

Vaccines. Vaccinate against hepatitis B, *Streptococcus pneumoniae*, and influenza.

HIV prevention. If available, ART should be given to the mother during pregnancy and to the infant after delivery to lower the chances that the infant will get HIV. (See the section on ART early in this appendix. See also Chapter 10, "Family counseling," for a further discussion of pregnancy in women with HIV.)

Pain

Some opportunistic infections, and HIV infection itself, can cause pain in a person's body. When people are in severe pain, it can be difficult for them to work, to care for themselves or others, or even to focus on basic activities. Besides treating the infection that is causing the pain, you may need to give medicines to stop the pain directly. No one needs to suffer with pain.

There are several common, easily available medicines that reduce pain, such as acetaminophen (or paracetamol, panadol, or Tylenol) or aspirin-like drugs (such as ibuprofen). However, severe pain may need opiates (such as codeine and morphine) and they are hard to get in many places because they often need a doctor's prescription. Opiates are very effective medicines, and can make a person's life much better. In many places, laws about who can give medicines are being changed so that nurses and other health workers can help treat pain with opiates. Talk to a doctor, nurse, or pharmacist about how to treat pain in a person with HIV.

Vaccines

Almost all of the vaccines given adults and children without HIV are recommended for people with HIV and for their household or family members. The exceptions are vaccines made with "live" viruses, which can cause disease in people with weak immune systems. Oral polio vaccine and bacillus Calmette-Guérin (BCG), both live vaccines, should generally not be given to people with AIDS or symptoms of HIV disease. In areas where TB is prevalent, however, BCG is recommended for infants who have no symptoms of HIV disease. Polio can spread from someone who has been vaccinated with the live virus to someone with HIV disease. For this reason, inactivated polio vaccine (IPV) is recommended not only for people with HIV but for their household members. Measles-mumps-rubella (MMR), although a live vaccine, should be given, as it has been shown not to cause any more problems in people with HIV than those without HIV. With a few exceptions, then, children and adults with HIV should be given the usual vaccines to protect them from illness.

Recommended vaccines for people with HIV	
Vaccine	Give to people with HIV?
Diphtheria-tetanus-pertussis (DTP)	yes
Oral polio vaccine (OPV)	no
Inactivated polio vaccine (IPV)	yes
Measles-mumps-rubella (MMR)	yes
Hemophilus influenzae type b conjugate	yes
Pneumococcal polysaccharide	yes
Influenza	yes
Bacillus Calmette-Guérin (BCG)*	no
Hepatitis B	yes

*Do not give to adults or children, or infants with symptoms of HIV infection. In areas of high prevalence of TB, infants may be vaccinated if they do not have symptoms of HIV disease.

Glossary

abortion. The ending of pregnancy before the fetus is able to live outside the woman.

acid-fast bacillus. A bacterium that stains red with acid-fast stain (*Mycobacterium tuberculosis*, the cause of tuberculosis, is an acid-fast bacillus).

acupuncture. Traditional Asian health practice of placing thin needles into people's skin to treat illnesses.

AIDS (acquired immune deficiency syndrome or acquired immunodeficiency syndrome). A group of diseases caused by the human immunodeficiency virus, or HIV.

AIDS dementia. Changes in thinking, personality, and mood that occur in some people with HIV infection.

AIDS wasting syndrome. Loss of over 10% of body weight in people with AIDS; this is the reason AIDS has also been called "slim disease."

alcoholic. A person whose consumption of alcohol has negatively affected her or his life (*see* CAGE questions).

anal sex. When a man's penis is inside a woman's or man's anus.

anemia. A lower than normal number of red blood cells that causes people to feel tired and weak.

anergy. Loss of the immune system's ability to respond to certain antigens.

anonymous testing. Testing that does not use real names, so that the identity of a person receiving a test result is unknown.

antibiotic. A drug that kills microbes such as bacteria and fungi.

antibodies. Small proteins that are made by the body's immune system and that recognize and help get rid of foreign organisms and toxins.

antigen. Any foreign substance that causes an immune response.

antiretroviral drug. Any drug that works against a retrovirus. HIV is a retrovirus; zidovudine (AZT) is an antiretroviral drug.

anus. External opening of the bowel.

aphthous ulcers. Painful ulcers in the mouth or throat.

asymptomatic. Without symptoms.

bacillus Calmette-Guérin. A vaccine against tuberculosis.

bacterium. A one-celled microscopic organism. Many bacteria can cause disease.

biopsy. Surgical removal of a piece of tissue for examination under a microscope.

birth control. *See* contraceptive.

bisexual. Someone who is attracted to both men and women.

blood product. A part of the blood, such as red blood cells, platelets, plasma, or clotting factors.

blood transfusion. Giving blood by vein. Transfusions are often given during surgery or to children who have anemia from malaria.

body fluids. Any fluid in the body, for example, blood, urine, saliva, sputum, tears, breast milk, semen, and vaginal secretions.

bone marrow. Tissue in the center of bones that produces blood.

bronchoscopy. Examination of the lungs using a bronchoscope.

CAGE questions. Four questions that can be used to determine if someone may be an alcoholic (*see* Chapter 6).

candida. A fungus that commonly causes disease in the mouth and vagina.

casual contact. Non-intimate behavior such as working, eating, playing, or studying with other people.

CD4 cell. White blood cells that help coordinate the immune system. CD4 cells are infected by HIV.

CD4 cell count. A count of the number of T4 lymphocytes, which gives an idea of the strength of the immune system.

cell. The smallest working unit of a living organism.

cervical dysplasia. Abnormal appearance of the cells from a woman's cervix. Pap smears look for cervical dysplasia (*see* appendix).

cervix. The part of the uterus that is in the vagina.

coccidiomycosis. A disease caused by the fungus *Coccidioides.*

condom. A barrier that is put over the penis before sex to prevent pregnancy and the spread of sexually transmitted diseases (STDs) and HIV.

confidential testing. Keeping test results private so that only health workers and the person tested know the results.

contraceptive. A product that prevents pregnancy; types include condoms, the Pill, the diaphragm, Depo-Provera, and the intrauterine device (IUD).

cryptococcal meningitis. An illness caused by infection of the covering of the brain with the fungus *Cryptococcus neoformans.*

cutaneous. Having to do with the skin.

cytomegalovirus (CMV). A type of herpes virus that often causes disease in people with damaged immune systems.

dehydration. The condition of a person's body having less water than is necessary to be healthy. Severe diarrhea can lead to dehydration.

DNA (deoxyribonucleic acid). A substance found in the nucleus of all cells that is the basic component of genes.

drug injector. Someone who injects drugs; generally used in this book to mean someone who injects illegal drugs such as heroin, cocaine, or amphetamines.

ELISA (enzyme-linked immunosorbent assay). A common test for HIV that looks for antibodies to the virus in a person's blood. Also called EIA.

encephalopathy. Damage to the brain.

epidemic. A higher rate of disease in a community than is expected—usually used to describe infectious diseases.

epidemiology. The study of diseases in populations or communities.

false negative. When a test is negative but a person does have the disease that is being tested for.

false positive. When a test is positive but a person does not have the disease that is being tested for.

family planning. Controlling the number and timing of children. Couples may use abstinence or contraceptives to plan their families.

gastrointestinal. Relating to the mouth, throat, esophagus, stomach, intestines, liver, gallbladder, or pancreas.

gay. Someone attracted to people of the same sex; homosexual.

gene. Unit of DNA that carries information for making proteins and that determines all inherited traits, such as skin color, eye color, and height.

hairy leukoplakia. A white, raised plaque usually found on the side of the tongue.

hemophilia. A disease caused by the lack of a special part of the blood (clotting factor) that allows a person to stop bleeding.

hepatitis. Inflammation of the liver; usually caused by viruses, alcohol, or drugs.

herpes simplex I and II. Viruses that cause cold sores, genital sores, and sometimes encephalitis.

herpes zoster (shingles). Painful blisters on the skin common in people with weakened immune systems; caused by the *Varicella zoster* virus (chicken pox virus).

heterosexual. Someone attracted to people of the opposite sex.

histoplasmosis. A infection, usually of the lungs, caused by the fungus *Histoplasma capsulatum.*

HIV. Human immunodeficiency virus, the virus that causes AIDS.

HIV-sheltered relationship. A sexual relationship in which no one has HIV infection, and no one participates in behaviors that would put her or him at risk for HIV.

homosexual. Someone attracted to people of the same sex.

human papillomavirus. A virus that causes genital warts and cervical cancer; HPV.

IDU. Injection drug user; also known as a drug injector or intravenous drug user (IVDU). Someone who injects drugs in order to become intoxicated.

IM. *See* intramuscular.

immune system. The body's defense against foreign organisms and substances.

immunity. Resistance to a specific disease.

incidence. The number of new cases of a disease in a community or population over a period of time, usually one year.

incubation period. Time between infection and the first symptoms of disease.

industrialized nations. Countries whose economies are based on manufacturing. Most of the countries in Europe and North America are industrialized.

influenza (flu). A disease of the throat and lungs caused by a virus.

informed consent. Agreement to have a test or procedure after being told the risks and benefits.

injectionist. A person who gives medicines by needle to people outside of a health clinic or hospital.

intramuscular (IM). Injected directly into the muscle.

intravenous (IV). Injected inside a vein.

intravenous needles. Hollow needles used to give drugs or blood, or remove body fluids.

IV. *See* intravenous.

Kaposi's sarcoma. A cancer caused by herpesvirus 8; it is usually characterized by red-purple lesions on the skin or internal organs.

lesbian. A woman who is attracted to other women.

lesion. An abnormal change in tissue caused by disease or injury.

leukopenia. Low white blood cell count.

lumbar puncture. A procedure in which a needle is used to take spinal fluid from the lower back.

lymphadenopathy. Abnormal swelling of the lymph nodes.

lymphocyte. A type of white blood cell.

lymphoma. A cancer of the immune system.

mandatory testing. Required testing.

masturbation. Touching of one's own genitals for sexual pleasure.

menses. Monthly shedding of blood from the lining of the uterus—also called a "period" or "menstruation."

menstruation. *See* menses.

microbicide. A chemical that kills microbes such as bacteria and viruses.

monogamous. Having sexual relations with only one person.

mutual masturbation. When two people touch each other's genitals with their hands.

neonatal. Regarding the first four weeks of life.

neuropathy. Disorder of the nerves due to infection, disease, drugs, or injury.

nucleus. The central part of the cell that contains DNA.

nutrients. Substances that a person needs to stay healthy; for example, vitamins and minerals.

opportunistic infection. Illness caused by an organism that usually does not cause disease in a person with a normal immune system.

oral rehydration therapy (ORT). A solution of sugar, salts, and water that is used to replace fluid losses. ORT is especially useful for people with diarrhea.

oral sex. When a person's mouth touches a sexual partner's genitals.

organism. Any living thing.

outreach worker. A person who actively seeks out people in her or his community to provide them with education or health care.

parasite. An organism that must live off another organism to survive.

period. *See* menses.

placenta. Tissue within a woman's uterus (womb) that is created during pregnancy to feed the growing fetus.

platelets. Cells in the blood that are responsible for forming blood clots.

Pneumocystis jiroveci pneumonia (PCP). A lung infection that occurs in people with damaged immune systems.

PPD (purified protein derivative). A protein that is used in a skin test to see if a person has been infected with *Mycobacterium tuberculosis.*

prevalence. The proportion of people in a population who have a disease at a certain time.

prophylaxis. Measures taken to prevent disease.

protease inhibitors. Drugs that stop HIV from putting together copies of itself.

protein. A substance within all living organisms. Protein, along with carbohydrates, fats, vitamins, and minerals, is an essential part of a balanced diet.

pulmonary. Having to do with the lungs.

rectum. Part of the bowel before the anus.

retrovirus. A type of virus that must use reverse transcriptase to copy itself.

reverse transcriptase. A substance used by a retrovirus to make DNA from RNA in order to copy itself.

reverse transcriptase inhibitors. A group of drugs used to treat HIV infection that prevent the virus from making copies of itself. These medicines work by preventing the viruses' reverse transcriptase enzyme from working.

risk factor. A practice or characteristic that makes it more likely that a person will get or have a particular illness. For example, getting a blood transfusion from untested blood is a risk factor for HIV infection.

RNA. Genetic information used in cells to make proteins; some viruses, like HIV, use RNA instead of DNA to store genetic information.

role play. Practicing talking with others about difficult topics by acting out an imaginary situation.

safe sex. Sex that has no chance of spreading HIV, such as mutual masturbation.

safer sex. Sex that has little but some chance of spreading HIV, such as vaginal sex with a condom and oral sex.

scarification. The practice of using sharp instruments to cut a person's skin to leave a permanent scar.

semen. A sperm-containing fluid that comes from the penis during sex.

sensitivity. How well a test detects a disease.

seroconversion. Development of antibodies to a foreign organism or antigen in someone who did not have the antibodies before.

seronegative. When a person's blood is negative for antibodies to a particular infection, such as HIV.

seropositive. When a person's blood has antibodies to a particular infection, such as HIV.

serum. Yellow fluid that remains after blood has clotted.

sexual orientation. How a person identifies himself when talking about sexual relationships (as bisexual, homosexual, or heterosexual).

sexually transmitted disease (STD). A disease spread through sex; for example, gonorrhea, syphilis, and HIV.

sharps. Medical instruments that have sharp points or edges.

shingles. Painful skin blisters caused by the *Varicella zoster* virus (chicken pox virus).

shooting gallery. A place where drug injectors can rent syringes and inject drugs.

side effects. Unintended effects of a medicine, such as diarrhea.

slim disease. A term for AIDS used in some parts of Africa.

specificity. The percentage of times a test for a disease is negative when used on people who do not have the disease.

spermicide. A chemical that kills sperm. Spermicides, used with condoms or as a vaginal foam, can prevent pregnancy.

sterilize/sterilization. A method for cleaning needles and instruments that kills microbes and prevents the spread of disease.

symptoms. A noticeable change in a person's body that indicates the presence of a disease.

syndrome. A group of symptoms or diseases that are used to define an illness.

syphilis. An STD caused by the bacterium *Treponema pallidum.*

syringe. A tube attached to a hollow needle used to inject medicine or take a blood sample.

thrush. Mouth infection caused by the fungus *Candida albicans.*

true negative. When a test is negative and a person does not have the disease that is being tested for.

true positive. When a test is positive and a person does have the disease that is being tested for.

tuberculosis (TB). A disease caused by the bacterium *Mycobacterium tuberculosis.* Most people with TB have pneumonia, meningitis, or bone infection.

unsafe sex. Sex during which HIV is likely to be spread, such as vaginal or anal sex without a condom.

uterus. An organ within a woman's body that supports the growth of a fetus.

vaccine. A substance used to prevent infection by a disease-causing organism.

vaginal sex. When a man's penis is inside a woman's vagina.

vertical transmission. The spread of a disease from mother to baby.

virus. A small organism that needs other organisms' cells to reproduce.

wasting. *See* "AIDS wasting syndrome."

Western blot. A test for HIV that looks for specific antibodies against the virus.

Resources

We benefited from reading many books and articles while writing this book. Below are a few books that we found especially helpful. Many others may be available in your area.

Berer, M. *Women and HIV/AIDS: An International Resource Book.* London: Harper-Collins, Pandora Press, 1993.

Cohen, F. L., and J. D. Durham, eds. *Women, Children, and HIV/AIDS.* New York: Springer, 1993.

Cohen, P. T., M. A. Sande, and P. A. Volberding, eds. *The AIDS Knowledge Base.* Waltham, Mass.: Medical Publishing Group, 1990.

Cotton, D., and D. H. Watts, eds. *The Medical Management of AIDS in Women.* New York: Wyley-Liss, 1997.

Gordon, G., and T. Klouda. *Talking AIDS: A Guide for Community Work.* London: Macmillan Education, 1990.

Green, E. C. *AIDS and STDs in Africa: Bridging the Gap Between Traditional Healing and Modern Medicine.* Boulder, Colo.: Westview, 1994.

Hubley, J. *The AIDS Handbook: A Guide to the Understanding of AIDS and HIV.* London: Macmillan, 1990.

Mann, J., and D. Tarantola, eds. *AIDS in the World.* 2d ed. New York: Oxford University Press, 1996.

Peiperl, L. *Manual of HIV/AIDS Therapy.* Fountain Valley, Calif.: Current Clinical Strategies, 1995.

Pierce, C., and D. VanDeVeer. *AIDS: Ethics and Public Policy.* Belmont, Calif.: Wadsworth, 1988.

Piot, P., B. M. Kapita, E. N. Ngugi, J. M. Mann, R. Colebunders, and R. Wabitsch. *AIDS in Africa: A Manual for Physicians.* Geneva: World Health Organization, 1992.

Pohl, M., D. Kay, and D. Toft. *The Caregivers' Journey: When You Love Someone with AIDS.* New York: HarperCollins, 1991.

Sabatier, R. *Blaming Others: Prejudice, Race, and Worldwide AIDS.* London: Panos Institute, 1988.

———. *The Panos Dossier: AIDS and the Third World.* London: Panos Institute, 1988.

Sande, M. A., and P. A. Volberding, eds. *The Medical Management of AIDS.* Philadelphia, Pa.: W. B. Saunders, 1997.

Webman, D. M., and F. J. Alwon, eds. *Taking Action on AIDS: A Resource Book.* Needham, Mass.: Albert E. Trieschman Center, 1990.

Werner, D. *Where There Is No Doctor.* Berkeley, Calif.: Hesperian Foundation, 2006.

————. *Helping Health Workers Learn.* Berkeley, Calif.: Hesperian Foundation, 2005.
Williams, A. O. *AIDS: An African Perspective.* Boca Raton, Fla.: CRC Press, 1992.
World Health Organization. *W.H.O. Model Prescribing Information: Drugs Used in Sexually Transmitted Diseases and HIV Infection.* Geneva: World Health Organization, 1995.
————. *AIDS Prevention Through Health Promotion: Facing Sensitive Issues.* Geneva: World Health Organization, 1991.

Websites

New information about HIV/AIDS is being developed all the time. Some of the websites we have found most useful are listed here. All of them contain links to other websites as well:

www.aegis.com
AIDS Education Global Information System
One of the largest HIV/AIDS databases in the world, features the "Daily AIDS Briefing," current news about HIV/AIDS.

www.aidspan.org/globalfund/
AIDSPAN is a nongovernmental organization that monitors the Global Fund to Fight AIDS, Tuberculosis and Malaria.

www.cdc.gov
Centers for Disease Control and Prevention (United States government)
Contains articles, information and news about various health issues, including HIV/AIDS, in both English and Spanish.

www.hivdent.org
A site including treatment information and training resources for those who provide dental and oral health care to people with HIV.

www.unaids.org
Joint United Nations Program on HIV/AIDS
Contains articles, information and news about UN activities as they relate to the HIV/AIDS epidemic, statistics and other useful information.

www.who.org
World Health Organization
Contains articles, information and news about UN activities on international health issues and policy, in English, French and Spanish.

Index

rapid serologic test, 74, 75, 77, 79
rashes, 14–15, 184, 192, 193–94, 227
rate, 29
religion, 100–101, 136
retina, 200, 202
retroviruses, 6, 132, 185
reverse transcriptase, 9, 10
reverse transcriptase inhibitors, 10
risk of HIV: assessment, 2, 3, 31, 37, 43–49, 53–55, 57–58, 86–87, 115, 145, 172; and blood donation, 62–64; for health care workers, 66–68
ritonavir, 10
role plays, 42–43, 92, 124, 134–35, 136, 137
rural areas, HIV/AIDS in, 34, 35–36
Russia, 36, 99
Rwanda, 1, 19, 28

safer sex, 2, 39, 45, 46–53, 54, 86, 151; promotion of, 31, 146–47; talking about, 91, 96, 103, 111, 134, 136
safe sex, 44–45, 48, 54, 84
saliva, 44
Salmonella, 187, 211
sandflies, 196–97
saquinavir, 10
scabies, 198
scars and tatoos, 69, 140
scissors, 64
screening of blood donors, 26, 62, 63, 64, 82
seizures, 203, 204, 205
semen, 44, 45, 46–47, 49, 50, 51, 52, 55, 222
serum, 62, 75–77
sex: frequency of, 54; and health care workers, 105–6, 131; between men, 21, 22, 31, 33, 34, 35, 41, 46, 62, 86, 106–7, 146; between men and women, 20, 22, 31, 33, 35, 41, 102–3, 107, 109–10, 124, 134, 136; receptive/insertive partners during, 46; safer sex, 2, 31, 39, 45, 46–53, 53, 86, 91, 96, 103, 111, 134, 136, 146–47, 151; safe sex, 44–45, 48, 54, 84; spread of cytomegalovirus during, 200; spread of HIV during, 6, 20, 22, 24, 29, 31, 37, 40, 41–49, 151; talking about, 2, 3, 41, 42–44, 47, 48, 52, 103, 105–7, 126, 129, 131, 134, 136, 137, 168, 172; unsafe sex, 31, 37, 43–44, 45–46, 48, 49, 53, 57–58, 72, 78, 79, 82, 86, 96, 105–6, 107–8, 146; and women, 102–3; between women, 106–7
sexually transmitted diseases. *See* STDs
sexual orientation, 106–7, 136
sex workers, 24, 39, 106, 127, 128, 140, 152, 154;

as counselors, 141, 168, 175; HIV education for, 143, 144, 145, 146–47, 162–63, 166–67, 168, 172, 176, 177; HIV prevalence among, 27, 31, 36; HIV risk among, 41, 47, 54, 58, 62, 86, 87, 102, 145; in support groups, 118
sharps containers, 67–68, 72
Shigella, 211
shingles, 86, 198–99
sinus infections, 187, 215
skin diseases, 191–99
sleeping sickness, 204
sneezing, 6, 19, 29, 40
social/economic status, 98–100, 101–3, 104
sore throat, 14, 208, 227
South Africa, 34, 144
South Korea, 2, 19
spermicides, 52
spread of HIV, 2, 6–7, 19–23, 55; and behavior change, 7, 39, 53–55, 82–83, 145, 151; during blood transfusions, 6, 20, 22, 29, 31, 37; and casual contact, 29, 40; from mothers to babies, 6, 18, 20, 22, 29, 31–32, 33, 34, 37, 57, 59, 69–71, 80, 81, 83–84, 96, 110, 117, 140, 150, 152, 188; from needles and instruments, 6, 22, 27, 29, 31, 37, 40, 54, 55, 56–57, 58–61, 64–68, 86; during sex, 6, 20, 22, 24, 29, 31, 37, 40, 41–49, 151
Staphylococcus, 194, 195, 215
stavudine (d4T), 10, 186, 188
STDs, 221–30; and HIV, 2, 49, 50, 54, 86, 87, 92, 221, 222, 227, 230
Stevens-Johnson syndrome, 192, 193
Streptococcus, 194, 195, 215
stress, 204
suicide, 112, 116, 124, 155
sulfa-containing drugs, 193, 219, 220
sun sensitivity, 199
support groups, 114, 115, 119, 120, 124
surveillance, 26
swallowing, 18, 203, 205, 209, 210, 213
sweats, night, 13, 15, 18
Switzerland, 36
symptoms: of AIDS, 26, 84, 151–52, 187; of initial HIV infection, 2, 13–16, 18. *See also* tests for HIV
syphilis, 49, 50, 54, 86, 204, 227–28, 231

Tanzania, 49, 151
tattoos and scars, 69, 140
teaching techniques, 126, 128–37
teenagers, 108–9, 139, 144, 150, 156, 158, 161
television, 155, 158–60

Other books from Hesperian

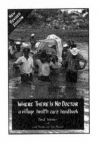

Where There Is No Doctor by David Werner with Carol Thuman and Jane Maxwell. Perhaps the most widely used health care manual in the world, this book provides vital, easily understood information on how to diagnose, treat, and prevent common diseases. Emphasis is placed on prevention, including cleanliness, diet, and vaccinations, as well as the active role people must take in their own health care. **512 pages**

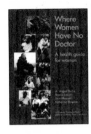

Where Women Have No Doctor by A. August Burns, Ronnie Lovich, Jane Maxwell, and Katharine Shapiro, combines self-help medical information with an understanding of the ways poverty, discrimination, and cultural beliefs limit women's health and access to care. An essential resource on the problems that affect women or that affect women differently from men. **584 pages**

A Book for Midwives by Susan Klein, Suellen Miller, and Fiona Thomson, completely revised in 2004, is for midwives, community health workers and anyone concerned about the health of women and babies in pregnancy, birth and beyond. An invaluable tool for training as well as a practical reference, it covers helping pregnant women stay healthy, care during and after birth, handling obstetric complications, breastfeeding, and includes expanded information for women's reproductive health care. **544 pages**

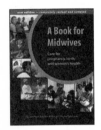

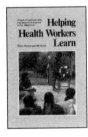

Helping Health Workers Learn by David Werner and Bill Bower. An indispensable resource for teaching about health, this heavily illustrated book presents strategies for effective community involvement through participatory education. Includes activities for mothers and children; pointers for using theater, flannel-boards, and other techniques; and ideas for producing low-cost teaching aids. **640 pages**

Helping Children Who Are Blind by Sandy Niemann and Namita Jacob, aids parents and other caregivers in helping blind children develop all their capabilities. Topics include: assessing what a child can see, preventing blindness, moving around safely, teaching common activities, and more. **192 pages.**

Where There Is No Dentist by Murray Dickson, shows how to care for the teeth and gums, and prevent tooth and gum problems through hygiene, nutrition, and education. Includes detailed, well illustrated information on using dental equipment, placing fillings, taking out teeth, and more. A new chapter includes material on HIV/AIDS and oral health. **237 pages.**

Helping Children Who Are Deaf by Sandy Neimann, Devorah Greenstein and Darlena David, helps parents and other caregivers build the communication skills of young children with difficulty hearing. Covers language development and how to foster communication through both sign and oral approaches, as well as assessing hearing loss, exploring causes of deafness, and more. **250 pages.**

Disabled Village Children by David Werner, covers most common disabilities of children. It gives suggestions for rehabilitation and explains how to make a variety of low-cost aids. Emphasis is placed on how to help disabled children find a role and be accepted in the community. **672 pages.**

1919 Addison St. #304, Berkeley, CA 94704 · USA · (510) 845-4507
www.hesperian.org · bookorders@hesperian.org